Contents

SECTION THREE: The future

About the editors

Robin Johnson read social science and philosophy at the University of Kent in the late 1960s, which was where he first became interested in concepts of mental health and mental illness. Discovering the therapeutic community approach, he worked and lived in a number of such communities in the 1970s, including the Henderson, one of the best known of all therapeutic communities. He then went on to train as a mental health social worker.

While working in a small multidisciplinary team in Nottingham, Robin became interested in the role of housing and homelessness services in working with some of the most vulnerable, chaotic and 'hard to reach' clients. In 2001, he set up the RJA consultancy practice to pursue an interest in research and development on mental health and housing. Since then, he has acted as an adviser to various government departments on innovative practice, emerging policy and the evidence base for service development.

Robin is now a member of the Royal College of Psychiatrists' Enabling Environments working group; joint editor of the journal *Housing, Care and Support*; and a visiting fellow at the Institute of Mental Health and the International Centre for Public Services Management at Nottingham Trent University. Robin was also an organiser of the local Café Scientifique for many years, where he says he gathered 'more perspectives on what it is to be a human being'.

Rex Haigh started his medical training in Cambridge where he studied social sciences and anti-psychiatry alongside anatomy, physiology, pathology and all the medical sciences. He then joined the Phoenix therapeutic community in Oxford for his psychiatric placement, and took and passed his medical finals in 1982.

After moving to Cornwall to train as a GP, and then back to Oxford to train as a psychiatrist, Rex was dismayed by the number of people let down by the mental health system and became a medical psychotherapist and a group analyst before working as a consultant psychotherapist for Winterbourne Therapeutic Community. While there, he helped refine and develop it into an effective and well-recognised personality disorder service.

In 2002, Rex helped to prepare the government's policy, Personality Disorder: No longer a diagnosis of exclusion, by organising the service user input. Since then he has been involved with both Emergence (formally known as Borderline UK) – as vice chair – and the National Personality Disorder as clinical advisor to the Department of Health's personality disorder work.

He leads the Royal College of Psychiatrists' Community of Communities and Enabling Environments quality networks, and has been a long-standing committee member and one time chair of the Association of Therapeutic Communities.

Introduction

Robin Johnson

Trauma in human experience

At the heart of this book is the subject of trauma, and the need for a better understanding of the nature and extent of trauma in human experience.

However, rather like the long aftermath of trauma itself, it does not stop there. In the course of exploring the nature of trauma and the challenges that psychological and emotional trauma presents, we aim to shed new light on psychological and social processes that reach into many, if not all, areas of modern social life.

The two editors have spent much of their careers working in community mental health services, and perhaps inevitably the psychiatric frame of reference colours and forms a constant backdrop to the themes that are highlighted here. Certainly we intend to argue that a better recognition of the nature and extent of trauma should play a pivotal role in reshaping our approach to the problems we see within contemporary psychiatry. It can also help us see these problems more clearly.

We wish to assert, however, a still more ambitious claim: that a better understanding of trauma is becoming the touchstone issue for a new and growing understanding of mental health, not just within the medical and allied professions but within society as a whole. We see this especially within the many other agencies that traumatised individuals will come into contact with over the course of their lives.

One of our central contentions is that much of this new understanding has in fact been evolving outside of the confines and frameworks of professional mental health services, and that those who do work in mental health may have as much to learn from examples of innovative practice in other areas – such as nurseries and schools, youth and community work, homelessness resettlement, occupational health and similar areas – as we do from colleagues within specialist mental health services.

This then becomes the springboard for a wider appreciation of the unseen role of trauma in the lives of troubled individuals, and of the work done by many individuals and many agencies to find a new and better way to respond.

This exploration of ways of working with trauma has at its heart the idea that the various groups, institutions and processes that make up our society – from families to schools, hospitals, workplaces and prisons, researchers and policy makers – may manage the emotional challenge well or badly, and when managed badly, they add to and compound the nature and complexity of the original trauma; they become part of the problem. An understanding of trauma in our lives cannot be separated from a broader questioning and critique of how well as a society we are doing in building emotional intelligence into the way we work.

Defining trauma

As the polymath and exuberant wordsmith Stephen Fry has observed, we tend to describe technical things in English by using words of Greek origin (Fry, 2007), which then allows us to describe the more personal and immediate aspects of life and the world around us in words of French or Anglo-Saxon rootstock. Thus, to be 'anaesthetised by trauma' has a more technical and medical connotation than to be 'numbed by shock', although the two phrases mean much the same thing.

By using the word trauma throughout this book we may therefore seem to be consigning and identifying the subject matter within a medical and scientific framework. We are, certainly, staking a claim that this is at least a relevant and helpful part of the story. However, this is not to forget that we are talking about the lived experience of traumatised individuals who are conflicted and struggling, and of the individuals around them who are equally struggling to help, or just to cope. We are suggesting that the terminology of trauma is helpful; we are not suggesting that it should take over from and replace an ordinary human understanding of each other.

We will therefore repeatedly shift the weight and language between the Greco-technical and the Anglo-human throughout this account, for effect. However, this is not simply a matter of writing style. Finding the right balance and constructive relationship between the medico-scientific description and the language of ordinary lives will be one of many recurring themes that run throughout the book.

Nevertheless, trauma – at least in the sense of psychological and emotional trauma – is not an easy or simple term to define in any precise and scientific way.

In physical care, trauma can be defined as *'a physical wound or injury, such as a fracture or blow'* (Martin, 2010), or only a little more loosely as *'a body wound or shock produced by sudden physical injury, as from violence or accident'* (Dictionary.com, 2012), where a 'shock' may be less precise or more pervasive in effect than an actual wound. All organs and bones are made of the same stuff, and with some allowances made for well-known factors such bone density etc, we can say with some confidence that a particular impact or stress will cause a particular damage. We can also say with reasonable confidence that a particular kind, place and degree of damage will account for a certain expected level of pain and distress. We must make allowances for the fact that different individuals may have different pain thresholds, distractions etc, but such subjective factors are at the periphery of the subject.

In physical health, then, we can move from the incident to the injury, the pain and the disability, with a confidence sufficient for most practical purposes.

In psychological and emotional trauma, by contrast, we are dealing not with an objective physical event and effect, but an experience. Psychological trauma is essentially a matter of how the individual has experienced an event. There may be huge differences in individual biography, in social support, in cultural references, and even in the personal meaning of an event that might affect whether, and by how much, any one individual might be traumatised by any one event. This fact makes it hard to define with any consistency or anything like precision what is a traumatising event, or a traumatising degree.

In the circumstances, a book on the effects of psychological and emotional trauma can take one or other of two approaches. One approach is to attempt to define trauma objectively and universally, by some agreed yardstick, with some kind of standard specification, perhaps notional but still hopefully useful.

The first problem with this approach is that no such agreed yardstick exists, and therefore most of the existing evidence for trauma may well have used some other threshold or specification. We will simply not know – or not without a great deal of enquiry – which existing studies we can use and include and which we cannot. A second equally salient concern is that through the relative arbitrariness of any particular specification we may exclude from view important studies that shed more light than the ones we allow.

The alternative is to take a much broader overview, and not attempt to pin ourselves to any particular – and perhaps premature – specification, other than to suggest that trauma is something that has overwhelmed the resources and capacity of the individual to cope, with damaging consequences. Perhaps now, almost by definition, we will know it by its effects.

In this book, for reasons that we hope will be apparent, it is the second course we have chosen. This will mean embracing the inevitable imprecision of a definition that is not objective and universal but a matter of individual biographies and circumstances, and prey to a wide range of subjective and wider social influences. If this does create dilemmas in attempting to trace the roots of trauma in any 'scientific' and defensively evidenced way, these are issues we will explore in one of the following chapters.

The relationship between stress and trauma

We also need to draw a boundary between trauma as such and that more ubiquitous phenomenon, 'stress'. Stress, however, has no more precise a definition. It has been variously described, for example, as:

- the non-specific response of the body to any demand for change
- the body's reaction to a change that requires a physical, mental or emotional adjustment or response
- the excitement, feeling of anxiety and/or physical tension that occurs when the demands placed on an individual exceed his or her ability to cope.

Stress in that sense may be a precursor to chronic stress ie. overload, or to extreme stress, as trauma. We might then locate psychological/emotional trauma as stress that surpasses a threshold of tolerance, to the point where it leaves lasting damage. This threshold definition is still not precise, however, as we now have good evidence that chronic stress without release also leaves damage. Trauma can also be seen (De Bellis, 2005) as an experience that induces an abnormally long stress response. The boundary between compound trauma and chronic stress may be particularly hard to define. It may be better to see stress and trauma as lying on a continuum, on which trauma is seen as arising from a more severe and shocking break with the individual's capacity to cope with challenging experiences.

Stress is certainly a widespread phenomenon in modern life. It is an issue that we can all recognise and so the concept of stress helps to make the links between our ordinary experience and the experiences of those who have had to cope with overwhelming stress.

We should also note that stress has a positive side: it equates with stimulation (Selye, 1975), and too little stress is perceived as boredom. There has been considerable attention paid lately to the management of stress, especially in workplaces, precisely in order that it should be motivating but not chronic or overwhelming. Research now emphasises that the more that workers are in control of their workload, have support from peers and have recognition of their efforts from senior staff, then the better they manage stress, and even thrive on it (Ryan & Deci, 2000). This is a theme that we will also see emerging from the various case studies of working with individuals with histories of trauma.

Nonetheless, it seems that the boundary between stress and trauma can at least be traced at a physiological level, in the way the brain functions. Mild to moderate stress will stimulate the growth of synaptic connectivity between neurons, as we learn to manage our situation, whereas under excess stress it appears that these systems shut down as more urgently self-protective responses take over.

There is, as we shall see, a growing school of thought that suggests that the careful re-introduction of stressful experience in controlled, manageable conditions may be the mechanism by which psychological therapies are effective (Cozolino, 2002; Folensbee, 2007).

A working definition of trauma

This then is the sense or meaning of the term trauma – psychological and emotional trauma – that will be used in this book: a trauma is any event or experience of sufficient force or magnitude that it overwhelms the capacity of the individual to absorb the experience and continue essentially unaffected, and which therefore results in a significant reduction or distortion of the individual's ability to carry on with normal behaviour and to function adequately in their lives.

It will be immediately apparent that this definition is still deeply problematic and indeed contentious. Who, after all, is to say what behaviour is normal, and what deviations from the norm are adaptive, and what dysfunctional? There is no universally agreed yardstick for what is acceptable or functional for a human being. This might therefore take us into some of the deeper and more philosophical questions over the nature of health as a normative state.

However, such questions must lie beyond the range of this book. For our purposes, we will adopt as the measure of functional health a more subtle, complex and possibly evasive definition: where the behaviour that an individual exhibits is deemed to need corrective action by other members of that society (with or without the formal intervention of the state and its institutions) then we will regard this as the key marker of psychologically traumatising experience and traumatised behaviour. In short, we will know trauma by its social consequences.

Admittedly this will bring into the definition, and therefore bring into the question, the nature of that society and its institutions, their tolerances and their capacity or will to muster a response. However, this is no bad thing, and it is the nature and scope of the societal reactions that we describe in this book – a somewhat circular definition, but one that we hope will at least give rise to interesting material, food for thought, and a coherent overview that will make all our examples legitimate.

In any case, until such time as a future book may attempt to unpick such philosophical complexities, this must be the boundary in practice of this exploration of managing trauma, and it will be sufficient for our purpose insofar as it is the actions of social institutions in managing trauma that are our primary concern.

The trauma continuum

We now need a term to describe the cumulative impact of a series of traumas. This is an all too common experience, compounding the impact of any original trauma with additional layers of complexity. If we can see such events as lying on a continuum of unfortunate experiences, then the natural term for the next level of difficulty might logically be that of 'complex' or 'compound' trauma.

Meanwhile, an accumulation of adverse experiences must eventually itself pass beyond some further threshold, and result in psychological and emotional disturbance that comes to the attention of those many agencies in society whose task is to correct behaviour that is becoming problematic. If this happens, the problematic experiences or disruptive impact may acquire a psychiatric label such as post-traumatic stress disorder (PTSD), conduct disorder or personality disorder (PD).

Hidden trauma, homelessness and the inspiration for this book

The ambition that motivates the writing of this handbook has been to attempt to see how far we might go in shedding new light on the phenomenon of PD and complex trauma, and how this may help us recognise the problems we face as a society and respond more constructively, and also to recognise constructive practice when we see it.

Ideas do not grow in a vacuum, and this book has its immediate origins in the work on which we, the editors and colleagues, were engaged, arguing for better recognition of the levels of psychological and emotional distress that homelessness services in the UK are encountering on a day-to-day basis.

The experience of homelessness always means more than simply not having a home. For some, a life on the open road may be an emblem of freedom. For others, it may be no more than a short but challenging episode in their lives. In some cases, a period of homelessness represents simply a brief episode, an unlucky break, or even a calculated but unsuccessful gamble on the part of some bright spark who takes a risk in seeking fame and fortune in another town or country. Clearly not all those who become homeless are in deep trouble.

For others, however, homelessness may be the end point of a downward spiral of complex social or mental health difficulties. Homelessness resettlement services are often working with those who have fallen through the various safety nets that support vulnerable people. They are managing not merely the practical assistance that individuals need to get themselves re-established in society, but also the emotional and social impact of such adverse circumstances.

In many cases they are working with individuals who have had a lifetime of adverse experience, compounding and entrenching any original abuse with further vulnerability and inability to cope, with many years and many layers of difficulties. Their problems are often the end of a long chain of conflicted relationships and rejections, and the often maladaptive responses that many people then adopt to fend off trust and the threat of more harm and hurt. This may then lead to relationships entangled in vehement ambivalence, until they eventually settle into what are called 'chaotic lives'.

These difficulties, which often go undiagnosed, may not amount to formal mental illness as such, at least in the narrowly-defined sense of psychosis, but there is plentiful indication of high levels of depression and anxiety, although it may be hard to distinguish such emotions from a natural reaction to such adverse circumstances.

We, the editors and colleagues, had been struck in particular by the fact that the often chaotic and self-defeating, distressed and distressing behaviour of such individuals bore all the hallmarks of what, in medical and psychiatric terms, would be called PD, and yet relatively few such individuals had any consistent involvement with mental health services. It seemed that there was a group of people with every indication of high levels of need who had been overlooked by psychiatry.

Rex Haigh's chapter, *Everybody's problem: the personality disorder dimension* (Chapter 1), shows that the underlying problems that the term PD rather clumsily describes are found among a far wider group than those in the psychiatric services with the diagnosis of PD formally given to them. A range of other cases of 'failures to respond to treatment' may therefore lie at the door of undiagnosed PD in both physical and mental health, as well as in society at large, in areas such as homelessness, the criminal justice system, youth and community work, occupational health, veteran servicemen and women, the emergency services and nurseries and schools.

The full extent of this issue only becomes apparent when we start to question what really underlies the diagnosis of PD, and at this point a considerable body of recent research, including both laboratory and clinical practice, starts to point towards early emotional or psychological trauma as the origin of much distress. A team at the Institute of Psychiatry (Nanni *et al*, 2011), for example, has recently marshalled the evidence and found that individuals who have suffered trauma and abuse in childhood are far more likely to present with depression in later life, and they will be those least able to respond to conventional treatment for depression. Again, the suggestion arises that trauma may underlie not just homelessness and PD, but far more.

The level of undiagnosed PD is therefore potentially quite serious. Equally serious, however, is the fact that there seemed to be little recognition – at least within mental health services – of the kind of work that the best of homelessness resettlement services were undertaking. This was especially striking because the profession of psychiatry is itself now trying hard to find new forms of treatment and new service models that will engage more effectively with the PD population that they do recognise – those who are failing to respond to standard treatments.

At a time when the Department of Health was keen to dispel what it described as 'therapeutic nihilism' and to promote innovation, we thought that there were lessons that might usefully be learnt by exploring how the best of homelessness resettlement services were approaching what seemed to be much the same issues. Indeed, as soon as we began to look outside clinical mental health care, it became increasingly apparent that there was a host of inventive services doing, in effect, preventive mental health work.

Our own investigations indicated that, for a full-blown textbook PD profile, it takes not just early emotional trauma, but a lifetime of compounding adverse events and mishandling. We were therefore inclined to explore as a useful framework the notion of complex or compound trauma, which many others have recently begun to propose as a more insightful description, and which was the language that was therefore used in the Department for Communities and Local Government's (CLG) guidance, which was published in 2010 along with the launch of the National Mental Health Development Unit (NMHDU).

From this starting point, the ambition developed to see how far we might go in shedding light on the phenomenon of PD and complex trauma, initially as seen from the perspective of, and using evidence from, homelessness. As a population who have fallen through the safety nets of social support, this is a useful working sample, and a good example of the extent to which a better recognition of PD or complex trauma – whichever formulation is more useful – can lead to new insights into effective ways to work with the underlying problems.

The Institute of Psychiatry study team, after their analysis of the relatively poor outcomes of otherwise effective orthodox treatments, had simply cautioned (King's Fund, 2011) that we may need to be sanguine about what these treatments can offer to those with histories of early trauma. Our own exploration suggests that there is good reason to be more optimistic – if we can only draw the right lessons from less conventional and less 'medical' practice.

The evidence of PD in homelessness

As Chapter 1 indicates, the diagnosis of PD is itself not without its problems, and indeed its critics. There is complexity and contention here, even before we begin tackling the additional complications of diagnosing PD or trauma in a setting already characterised by unstable, chaotic, stressful and dysfunctional life circumstances.

In addition to this complexity, homelessness itself cannot be treated as a single and homogeneous category of life experience. As already noted, homelessness may take different forms, and even different degrees. The emotional issues we might expect to find in a refuge for women escaping domestic violence will not be the same as those for homeless youngsters in a foyer, for street drinkers in night shelter, or rough sleepers in a bivouac in the woods.

Arriving at any reliable measure of the likely level of diagnosable PD in the homeless population therefore requires some careful sifting of the available evidence. It requires an element of interpretation of data that is sometimes patchy, sometimes ambiguous. Perhaps most of all, it involves an adequate understanding of the multiplicity of services and their different referral routes and criteria, and the data that they gather, each for their own purposes.

For example, in the UK we have an annual Survey of Needs and Provision (SNAP) (Homeless Link, 2008–2012) on the prevalence of mental health and other issues found in homelessness resettlement services ie. hostels and day centres. In these surveys, staff reported that 64% of projects identified some clients with PD, and 7% reported that more than half of all their service users did.

However, studies from Edinburgh (Murphy *et al,* 2002), Leeds (Middleton, 2008), London and Southampton (Maguire *et al,* 2010) suggest in fact a far higher identified prevalence of PD. For example, in the Edinburgh sample, 70% of service users had at least one diagnosable PD and 40% had two or more. In a study of a night shelter in New York (Connolly *et al*, 2008), the clinician researchers found very high rates of all PDs, and at least one Cluster A disorder (ie. the 'avoidant' and 'emotionally under-nourished') in 92% of their sample.

It may be significant that in each of the studies where higher levels of PD were reported, the homelessness resettlement service staff had received some training on the nature of PD. This variance in reported levels of PD may therefore reflect initially limited awareness or misapprehensions of PD. However, it may also suggest, perhaps, some reluctance by staff of these non-clinical services to ascribe such a stigmatised term unless the individual has a specific PD diagnosis. The low reported levels may therefore reflect markedly lower engagement of mental health services with this client group.

We may also note the relatively high recording in the SNAP surveys of 'complex needs'. This may be significant because in these surveys it is quite possible to indicate multiple needs by ticking a number of boxes. This therefore suggests that the term 'complex needs' is used to indicate not just a multiplicity of problems, which can be shown by ticking more boxes, but more complex emotional/behavioural issues – complex trauma.

If we take a step back from the specifically medical framework of PD diagnosis, symptom clusters etc, and look at the same evidence in more psychological terms, as difficulties experienced and the ways they may be expressed – if in short we do veer more towards the formulation of 'complex trauma' – then some of the difficulties in interpreting data are much reduced. We can readily recognise indications of deep-seated distress and chaotic lifestyles, with or without the additional challenge of formal diagnosis. We find, in short, ample evidence of trauma.

For example, there is evidence of a greater use of hospital accident and emergency units by homeless persons (Crisis, 2004). This may of course reflect the homeless person's lack of access to regular GP services. It may also be a measure of a higher level of physical injury through attacks, reflecting the higher risks entailed in a life on the streets as much as it does any personal characteristics of the victims of attack. However, that is simply to confirm that the situation of the homeless person is fraught with trauma.

There is also evidence of a higher incidence of suicide attempts (Haw *et al,* 2006; Public Health Agency of Canada, 2006), of deliberate self-harm (Cullum *et al*, 1995), and of PTSD (Taylor & Sharpe, 2008; Stewart *et al*, 2004; Gwadz *et al*, 2007), which does indicate higher levels of personal distress. The case studies of homelessness services' interventions that appear later in this collection and elsewhere (Cockersell, 2010; 2011; Whittington, 2011) certainly suggest that this profile is rife.

There is also good evidence of high levels of substance abuse among homeless persons. Substance abuse is known to be, at least statistically, 'associated with' PD, (Welch, 2002; Regier *et al*, 1990; Verheul, 2001; Seivewright & Daly, 1997). It is easy to see drug or alcohol use as a form of self-medication for the frustrations and disappointments of a life full of emotional difficulty. Even so, there is a need for caution: here in particular the dictum that 'correlation is not causation' is worth remembering. The relationship between substance abuse and PD may not be straightforward; it may be that becoming ensnared in drug use, or reliance on alcohol, brings out the worst in a personality previously only susceptible to disorder.

However, there are also known to be high levels of PD within the prison service (Singleton *et al,* 1998), and there are high levels of ex-offenders among homeless people (Social Exclusion Unit, 2002; Centre for Mental Health, 2011; Homeless Link, 2008–2012). It is often assumed that the PDs to be found in the prison population will be predominantly those of the 'antisocial' type (though as we shall see, there is some good reason to doubt this). These may not, however, be the ones that we find later in homelessness services; it may be the more chaotic, outwardly turbulent and dependent, who cannot settle. Some years ago a study by the Cabinet Office (Social Exclusion Unit, 2002) found that one third of prisoners were homeless at the time of conviction. This figure would seem to suggest a continuous flow of these most marginalised individuals between institutions that are merely holding them for a period.

For another perspective again, a recent literature review (Rees, 2009) of mental health problems among the single adult homeless population, commissioned by the charity Crisis, also suggests a high level of 'mental health problems' of all kinds, among other issues. Both the SNAP and Crisis studies estimate that the prevalence of common mental health problems is over twice as high, and of psychosis four to 15 times as high, among the homeless population compared to the general population.

This again might suggest at least a comparably heightened prevalence of other major mental health problems such as PD among the homeless population. (The Crisis literature review itself concluded that the evidence suggested a high prevalence of PD, though the actual numbers might be hard to quantify.) And finally, if it is true, as some estimates have found, that as many as 10–14% of the population as a whole have personality difficulties tantamount to PD (Torgersen *et al*, 2001), then to expect a still higher proportion within homelessness services may seem less of a wild claim.

Taken together, these many studies and statistics suggest, at the very least, a likelihood of significantly higher level of diagnosable PD among the single adult homeless population. However, they also suggest that there may be an unclear boundary between individuals' presentations of distress. While this may reflect imprecision in the survey, assessment or other measurements, it may also indicate that among the homeless population, clear-cut distinctions between diagnostic concepts are less applicable. Episodes of homelessness may then be seen as only one subset of adverse outcomes for those with a potential diagnosis of PD, but the issues involved in tracing the nature and numbers here may also shed useful light on similar problems in identifying the nature and course of PD – or complex trauma – elsewhere.

We have therefore suggested that, taken together, these complex presentations are most usefully conceptualised as indicative of a single broad syndrome of complex trauma. We have taken this as the unifying framework for this overview, rather than any current and prematurely narrow medico-diagnostic formulations. It is this broader concept and its links with the narrower diagnostic formulations of PD that the introductory chapters explore.

CLG guidance

If rates of PD in the population at large may be as high as 10 or 14% (Torgersen *et al*, 2001), then it is also clear that what is being studied and assessed here is not simply the rates of antisocial PD, which is the form of PD that has attracted most attention in the media. There are other ways of struggling emotionally, and Chapter 1 explores the many faces of dysfunctional personality.

When you look more closely, the description of PD in the recent CLG and NMHDU homelessness guidance (CLG/NMHDU, 2010) is radically different from the media stereotype of the deranged axe man and cold-blooded killer.

This greater understanding of the nature of PD is also reflected in the assessment practice of the homelessness outreach teams referred to in the guidance. One of the practice examples that the guidance praises is an assessment tool – it is quoted in full in the guidance – that was developed by the specialist PD service in Leeds, which works closely with local homelessness outreach services. The language of their questions indicates their very different approach:

- How much does the client reflect on their actions and consider how effective their plans have been?
- How much do they learn from experience? (Do they adjust their plans based on past experiences?)
- What is the client like at asking for, and co-operating with, help?
- In what ways does the client help others?
- What conflicts crop up for the client? (What does the client get cross about?)
- What is the client like at listening to and understanding others? (What are they like at communicating?)

- Does the client think other people listen to and understand them?
- What does the client get anxious, fearful or worried about?
- How does the client react when anxious?
- What causes the client to become low in mood or fed up?
- What activities does the client enjoy doing?

The range of difficulties in relationships that they describe will be familiar to some degree to us all. That is perhaps the key point: we can all recognise these issues because they are about being human, and struggling to cope. There is certainly nothing overly medical in this. Still, *'this guide deliberately tries'*, it says, *'to avoid the polarised argument about homelessness being either the fault of the individual or the fault of society, but rather sees homelessness as resulting from an interaction of the two'* (CLG/NMHDU, 2010).

Whether that in itself is enough to forestall future pigeon-holing of homeless people remains to be seen. There is always the risk that some people will complain that any use of medical or even psychological terms means medicalising what is really a social problem. As a result, we are still more strongly inclined to support the emergence of an alternative way of conceptualising PD, as complex trauma.

Nevertheless, if such individuals were to come to the attention of the psychiatric services, they would in all likelihood be given a diagnosis of PD. In truth, however, there would be little to be gained from this. In most parts of the country, specialist mental health services had neither the skills nor the inclination to help with such entrenched problems.

In fact, the CLG/NMHDU homelessness guidance suggests that the term 'personality disorder' itself may not be much help in the homelessness world. However, this is only partly because of the persisting stigma and 'therapeutic nihilism' that goes with the term. The other reason is that the diagnosis rests, by implication, most of the problem with the individual. Instead, the guidance suggests, we have to consider how poor some services are at recognising the real emotional needs underlying chaotic behaviour, and the equally chaotic way services in some areas simply do not 'join up' and gear up to manage more challenging behaviour (Cabinet Office, 2006).

Yet in practice these problems are typically being dealt with by services other than the mental health services. Despite the evident value of the PD demonstration pilots in creating new specialist services within the NHS, which Rex Haigh's paper in Chapter 1 briefly describes, it would be as or more constructive in future for psychologically skilled health and social work staff to provide a supportive role to those other agencies in society that may well be dealing with many of the same underlying problems.

For this, we will need a broader overview, and perhaps also a new vocabulary to describe the issues being dealt with, including those issues being managed in more preventive services that are working with the very beginnings of trauma, before the full complexity of compound trauma has taken root. We must also consider the work of other services, further down the line, attempting to undo the damage or prevent further harm. For this, we need to explore where such work is currently being done and what we might learn from these different fields – to join the dots as it were – and that is the focus of Section two of this book.

Joining the dots

There seems to be a growing tendency within many areas of our busy organisational lives to say, in effect, 'We really must focus on our own area of interest and expertise; we simply don't have the time to talk to others and to learn from their experience.'

This tendency now seems particularly marked throughout frontline public services of all kinds. One of the commonest – and certainly the saddest – refrains in all inquiries after a death or serious incident is that 'agencies failed to communicate with each other'.

More worrying still, that same tendency is even more pronounced in vocational education. In the working world outside there may now be constant encouragement to work more holistically, to collaborate, to form partnerships and work across agency 'silo' boundaries. In the university and training system, however, we still focus on teaching the core skills of each profession as if in parallel universes. Under the grim pressures of exam stress, students want to know only what they need to know to get through the next exam; all else must wait.

What is true of vocational learning is equally true of research, and each area of expertise now has its own assumptions and its own evidence base. The caustic comment that an expert is someone who knows more and more about less and less has particular force within academia. What is regarded as good evidence in one field is ignored or dismissed in another and we no longer thrash out fundamental ideas about human nature.

This book is dedicated to the opposite view. We believe that there are as many striking similarities as there are differences in the underlying nature of the problems that we tackle, each in our different areas. Across a wide range of what we propose to call 'social practice' – that is, all areas of civil society, of life and work where we are dealing with 'social' issues in a broad sense – we suggest that services have much in common and a great deal to learn from each other.

In innovative practice in particular there is a common thread, and we suspect that all pioneering spirits have the most to learn from each other. Section two of this book, we hope, illustrates these continuities with examples of services and approaches from a wide range of innovators – whether individuals or, more commonly, agencies, services and teams.

Reading this book

Not all readers of this book need to read, or will be equally interested in, all of its sections and chapters – especially in the central section, where we introduce innovative practice in specific fields. It will probably always be tempting to focus first on the fields we know or that most resemble our own.

However, this book is not intended as a set text or as required reading on any particular course. It is intended instead as a resource to stimulate thinking for all those who are interested to see what similarities there are between different approaches and areas, and what we can take from elsewhere and apply in our own agencies.

Little in this book may be entirely new or surprising, therefore. Everything in it is obvious to someone. Some of it, we hope, is obvious to everyone. It is not our intention to unveil dramatic new knowledge, but rather to show in a different light the things we always knew – but perhaps did not always know we knew. If then at times we speak boldly of a new synthesis, it is more a matter of re-arranging and reconciling, of reflecting back.

Above all else – and however useful some snippets of scientific discovery or case studies of inspirational practice may be – it is reflective practice, shared action learning, which we see as the key. For all that individuals may learn or teach, it is when we go forward together that we make real progress.

Section one

The nature of trauma

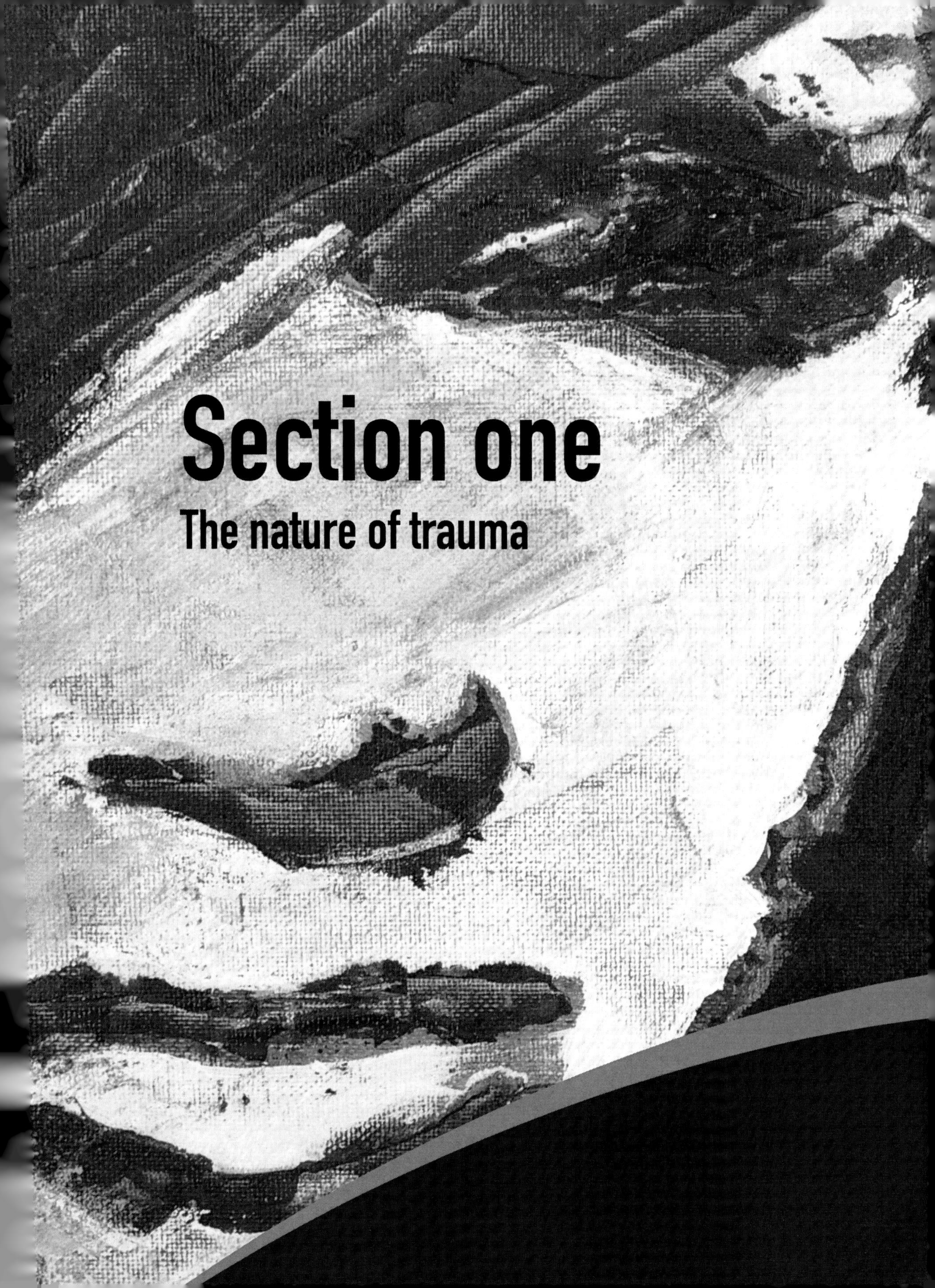

Section one:

The nature of trauma

Introduction

In this first section we will explore and hold up to critical scrutiny new insights into the nature of trauma and its impact throughout life, both on the individuals who have experienced major trauma, and on others around them with whom these individuals then interact. These new insights come from three main sources.

First, they come from the dialogue between psychiatric practice and the emerging discipline of epidemiology, which is beginning to show us facts about the extent and the concentrations of poor health, and especially poor mental health, in the community at large. In this section we will consider new evidence suggesting that compound, developmental trauma – trauma in its broadest sense – is far more widespread and pervasive than previously thought, not solely in homelessness services but in the population as a whole. We will explore the way traumatic experiences may later be expressed and re-enacted through clusters of problematic behaviour, emotions and thoughts.

We will outline the radical rethink on the nature of personality disorder (PD) and of underlying personality problems, and explore the new approaches that are being developed through the pilot site services developed originally for the Department of Health by the National Institute for Mental Health in England. Under the claim that PD is 'everybody's problem', we will suggest that any new agenda for 'happiness' or 'well-being' has to tackle not merely depression and anxiety – the so-called 'common mental health problems' that we now all freely talk about – but some much deeper, harder issues that have been hidden from view for too long.

Second, there are new insights that come from contemporary neuroscience, showing relationships between the human brain and human experience that shed a very different light on past models of human nature, and of psychopathology. These new findings, made possible by enormous advances in the technologies of neuro-imaging, are also complemented and enriched by new developments in our understanding of evolution and human development, both as a species and as individuals.

From this we will derive an approach to trauma that is significantly different in key respects from the model of trauma that has dominated clinical and specialist medical services: the biomedical model, which still pervades our thinking, especially in research. Rather than adopting the standard biomedical assumption of illness or pathology, we suggest a perspective that regards developmental diversity and the risks that it entails as part of life, and part of the human condition.

Third, there are useful insights that come from more systemic approaches – those that attempt to understand the interlocking complexities of the social world as a whole, rather than breaking it into discrete fragments and compartmentalising problems to make them manageable. We will take a fresh look at some ideas on social systems that have helped in the past to shed light on how organisations function in the face of an onslaught of emotional pressures that they are poorly equipped to cope with.

We will highlight the need to address not merely the characteristics and training needs of individual staff, but to look at how organisations themselves function, for good or ill. This is a theme that also runs through many of the examples in Section two of the book, and we return to explore this in more practical ways in the third and final section.

But first, at this exploratory stage in the development of this new framework, it may be helpful to revisit the original basis of the diagnosis of PD within medicine. We do so not because the problems necessarily lie within the framework of medicine – as we shall see, the more dynamic and less diagnosis-based formulations of clinical psychology and psychotherapy may well offer a better match for the presentations seen by other agencies – but in order to begin to see how different presentations of distress or dysfunctional behaviour have been managed and conceptualised in different ways by different sectors in society.

To begin, we must first consider the way that medicine has identified these problems – when it does so at all – in terms of PD.

Chapter 1

Everybody's problem:

the personality disorder dimension

Rex Haigh

When human development is disturbed, the psychological, social and economic consequences can reach into every area of an individual's personal and social world, resulting in alienated and chaotic lives and with repercussions throughout their communities. The causes of these disruptions may arise from a whole range of physical, environmental, psychological, social and economic factors, from an unlucky genetic inheritance to a difficult birth, child abuse, inadequate parenting, failed attachment, trauma or emotional deprivation, rejection and exclusion.

Recent studies, such as Wilkinson's (2006) and Marmot's (2009) work, now suggest that economic inequality underlies many of the persistent health problems of modern societies, and material poverty is clearly a factor in the struggle for a satisfactory life. However, poverty of expectations, which can leave individuals feeling powerless to have any impact on the world in which they live, is deeply implicated in the emerging account. Differences in class and educational advantage may confer some protection, as do strong constitutions or a range of other poorly understood protective factors that may be sufficient to enable an individual to withstand the impact of these environmental failures and emerge from their early experience to live what appear to be thriving and healthy lives.

However, very many with more severe problems end up in a situation where they are excluded from mainstream society, rejected by those who might be able to help them and destined to live lives of unremitting frustration, without the happiness and fulfilment that most of us would expect for ourselves and our families. These individuals, and often their families, have little psychological sense of their place among others or where they fit into society. School, working lives and almost any pro-social relationships are difficult or impossible to establish and sustain. They come to experience the world as a hostile, unhelpful, threatening or undermining environment, some living in a marginalised underclass with high levels of substance misuse, self-harm and criminality, and suffering severe, enduring and disabling mental distress. People in this situation will often use a considerable range of statutory services to little benefit.

This is the reality of personality disorder (PD).

If we are to believe the account that we find in the media, those with PD are the cold, dangerous and devious villains of countless B-movie dramas. Hollywood has an endless appetite for the sensational and for the exploitation of stereotypical villainy for cheap plots with plenty of guaranteed drama and no messy introspection or personal history to confuse our sympathies. By contrast, deep anguish and disturbed behaviour (which may well indicate underlying PD) is generally portrayed either with sympathetic understanding or with clinical alienation – neither of which ever hint at the diagnosis or the extraordinary ubiquity of its prevalence.

However, it is not just Hollywood. The mainstream news media too may rely on a thrill and hint of demonology for good readable copy. Even sober and respectable science programmes readily fall prey to the temptation to jazz up a technical discussion of some recent neuroscience finding with an intro of sound clips from Hitchcock's *Psycho*, and so wrongly render it well out of the normal range of human experience (Nature, 2010).

Only a minority of people with these problems will receive the PD diagnosis and then gain access to appropriate intervention services. The majority will receive an ambiguous and often prejudicial perception of their difficulties and will be more likely to meet a range of unsatisfactory public service responses. Depending on the immediate presenting difficulty, this response will often be inconsistent and have little relevance to the core psychosocial problem faced by individuals who are trapped in the experience of a failing relationship – not just in one area of their lives, but with the world around them, and even more fundamentally, with themselves.

People who suffer in these ways often do so silently, without getting any effective help and often feeling guilty or ashamed of how they 'are'. Often they do not even know that their problem is shared by others, and they can become very isolated and lonely. In fact, these problems are very common and are becoming increasingly recognised. The reason people behave the way they do, and have the difficult relationships they do, is usually in an effort to deal with intolerable emotions and to try and cope with them. However, their actions often do not help enough and they can make matters worse.

Very commonly these 'behaviours' can be confusing and upsetting, and this is as true for the people themselves as for those around them. This is because there is a lack of information and understanding about how these things arise, unwillingness to think and talk about them, and little knowledge about what can be done to support someone in this sort of emotional turmoil. The world needs to change in its attitude towards and understanding of such people if the sufferers are themselves going to be able to change.

What is a rational though largely unconscious reaction to intolerable circumstances gives justice to the proposition that in fact it is the world that is maladjusted not just those with PD. RD Laing (1966; 1967) said much the same for schizophrenia. His contribution to mainstream psychiatry was subsequently sidelined by pharmacology (as well as his own later and over-zealous efforts to celebrate what were manifestly painful and distressing symptoms of psychosis). However, in the age of the internet and service user empowerment it will be more difficult to put the genie of needing to change the establishment view of mental health back into the bottle.

A recent example comes from the government's most rigorous arbiter of clinically proven practice, the National Institute of Clinical Excellence (NICE). Among several other recommendations in its 2009 guidelines for treating Borderline Personality Disorder (BPD), two of its conclusions fly directly in the face of most contemporary clinical practice:

- stop using medication
- use long-term psychotherapy.

Although medication is often the easiest route to offer some amelioration, and although 'poly-pharmacy' (the prescription of several different types of medication, often at high dose, and generally accumulated over several years in response to a lack of substantial improvement) is the commonest professional response, recent research has failed to show that it offers any long-term help.

NICE declared that medication should only be used for specific indications and for time-limited periods. In the NHS, psychological treatment often helps, and this may take different forms. However, short-term 'quick fix' treatments and therapies are rarely very much help, and again the NICE investigation confirmed this. NICE stated in the guidelines that treatment needs to establish prior conditions such as hope and optimism, and take place over months and years rather than weeks.

Some mainstream psychiatric services are good at helping people with these problems, but because the number of people affected has only recently been recognised and reached wider awareness, many mental health staff do not yet have good training to deal with it. If it is government policy to hold that there is 'no health without mental health' (RCP, 2010), this vast burden of morbidity needs to be addressed. This was the task of the Department of Health's National Personality Disorder Development Programme, until the demise of its central co-ordination in April 2011. The national Knowledge and Understanding Framework (KUF) continues to be implemented throughout England.

What's in a name?

What exactly is PD?

First, most people are agreed that personality disorder is a terrible term, and nobody likes it very much. It is generally seen as pejorative and blaming. For many years it was associated with what the Department of Health has criticised as 'therapeutic nihilism' – a grim prognosis and a general sense that these are people who cannot be helped, as if the fact that we had found few effective treatments is a problem to blame on the sufferer.

However, for the moment at least, PD is the word we use to cover a series of problems that need some kind of description. PD, or whatever term we might use instead, is about a failure of satisfactory emotional development. It is serious, and it is everywhere.

PD problems are primarily reflected in the conduct of relationships – relationships with the world in general, including one's relationship with oneself. (In the rather obscure and technical language of psychodynamics, their object relations are somehow disturbed.) This failure to relate to both self and others in a healthy way is what PD is all about. As a condition it is responsible for pervasive, chaotic and expensive effects on society, which cross many organisations, services and systems.

PD lies at the root of many problems – a considerable proportion of mental ill-health, social exclusion, educational failure, drug and alcohol abuse, antisocial behaviour, criminality, bullying, disrespect, abuse of power, unemployability, and unnecessary conflict in social situations can all often be laid at its door. It is 'everybody's problem'.

However, for the individual with PD, their own experience of life and relationships – though it may fluctuate in intensity over time – is commonly that of lifelong suffering of rejection, anguish and alienation from the rest of the world. The 'typical' person with PD is not calculating, cold and calm under pressure. On the contrary, he or she is struggling with a chaotic life, and often doing so in silent desperation.

Others close to them, perhaps with responsibilities as carers, may be worried about particular behaviour, including:

- self-harming behaviour
- drinking unsafe amounts of alcohol
- taking illegal drugs regularly, excessively or irresponsibly
- misusing prescribed medications (or those available over the counter at pharmacies)
- impulsive and reckless actions that could have serious consequences, such as driving too fast or having unsafe sex
- chaotic eating patterns, such as bingeing, vomiting, abusing laxatives or continuously eating too much.

It is easier to see these problems from the outside. However, here are some examples of things that some people with PD might recognise in or say about themselves:

- I never keep friends very long
- I cannot hold down a job
- I feel isolated and lonely
- I experience violent intimate relationships, often repeatedly
- I am oversensitive to criticism

- I am argumentative with people in authority
- I feel very abandoned when left alone or when people leave
- I am unable to cope with making any decisions without help
- I am often switching between loving and hating family members.

As we might expect for something so pervasive, PD comes with many other names, often quite negative in implication. In different contexts, people with PD may be known or described as:

- complex cases
- heart-sink patients
- fat-file cases
- multi-agency families
- suffering medically unexplained symptoms
- bipolar, schizophreniform
- suffering from complex or chronic post-traumatic stress disorder.

The underlying problems come with many different descriptions too. They might be described as:

- environmental failure
- parenting failure
- disrupted human development
- attachment disorder
- complex trauma
- lifelong emotional difficulty
- lack of emotional intelligence.

However, those who come to the attention of the health services and psychiatry may increasingly expect to get a PD diagnosis. Although the ethics and mechanisms of 'the act of diagnosis' are themselves complex (for example, how long a clinician should personally know a patient before entering such a diagnosis onto a computer system where it may hamper future care by others), arriving at a diagnosis by careful interview is genuinely difficult. Indeed, for research purposes, the interviews themselves are closely manualised and interviewers require training and rehearsal with videos to ensure they are reliably reporting the diagnoses.

PD in psychiatric terms

The results of these structured interviews or other diagnostic processes are clustered and categorised by modern psychiatry into the definitive diagnostic categories as recognised by either the World Health Organization (and classified into the International Classification of Diseases (ICD)) or the American Psychiatric Association (and classified into the Diagnostic and Statistical Manual (DSM)). Both systems are in common use in the UK and are broadly similar for PD although the DSM is almost always used for research.

In version 4 of the DSM IV-TR (fourth edition, text revision), the 10 diagnoses (diagnostic categories) are divided into three clusters. Some clinicians find the cluster system more useful than the individual categories, either for giving clues about what sort of background somebody has had, or for assessing severity. The clusters are called A, B and C.

Cluster A

Cluster A is called 'odd or eccentric', and as a broad generalisation it includes people who are diagnosable in this way who usually 'live in their own world', and do not often seek help for their relationship problems. The three diagnoses are:

- paranoid (predominantly suspicious of others)
- schizoid (predominantly cut off from and uninvolved with others)
- schizotypal (predominantly superstitious and believing odd things).

This has been seen as the 'cold cluster' – describing a detached and 'cut off' quality in relating to others. Indeed, attachment theory is similar in its description of the type of insecurity known as 'avoidant attachment'. Clinically, we often see it arising from 'emotional undernourishment', or lack of love, or frank neglect.

Cluster B

Cluster B is called 'dramatic and erratic', and people who fall into one of these categories often have emotions that are 'all over the place'. The four diagnoses are:

- borderline (unstable in mood, sense of self and behaviour)
- narcissistic (sustaining self-image by exaggeration)
- histrionic (given to overly dramatic displays of emotion)
- antisocial (lack of empathy and remorse).

This has been called the 'hot cluster', at least within mental health services, as people with these problems often cause much heat in their relationships. Attachment theory – one of the most useful perspectives in psychology developed in recent years – suggests similarities to the type of insecurity in children known as 'disorganised attachment', at least for borderline PD. Clinically, we often see borderline PD linked with severe inconsistencies in childhood, frequently including sexual abuse. Antisocial type PD can often be linked to histories of neglect and physical violence.

Cluster C

Cluster C is called 'anxious and fearful', and people who are diagnosable in this way often do not get referred for specialist treatment as they are dealt with in primary care. The three diagnoses are:

- obsessive-compulsive (with great anxiety if things are not 'just right')
- dependent (unable to make decisions alone, and very anxious about it)
- avoidant (very anxious about relating to others but wanting to – unlike schizoid).

People with diagnoses in this cluster frequently spend the majority of their waking life at home, often feeling anxious, and unable to leave it without feeling extremely uncomfortable. Attachment theory suggests similarities to the type of insecurity known as 'anxious attachment'. Clinically, it can be understood most commonly as a failure to mentally establish a 'secure base' from which to explore and establish an independent sense of safety.

Note, however, that these diagnoses are frequently overlapping, and most people with severe problems have a mixture of features from each sub-type, and from each cluster. Although some researchers – and some service users – find it useful to make claims such as 'They have/I have been diagnosed with six PDs', such statements have little clinical relevance. Other researchers have described severity as a combination of the number of individual categories and the number of clusters covered, but again, any definite clinical relevance of this has not been proven. Many clinicians therefore do not find the separate categories of PD types very useful.

Note also that many service users also tend to reject the term PD – partly fearing the stigma and 'therapeutic nihilism', partly feeling that they have been categorised but not understood, and partly fearing that the diagnosis is in effect an accusation that the whole of their personality is to blame. With PD, unlike other psychiatric conditions, you do not have symptoms that are distinct from the 'real' or 'inner' you: there is nowhere you can hide.

Psychotherapists and psychologists meanwhile, who have often been the healthcare professionals most willing to get to the bottom of the PD diagnosis and the problems it describes, tend to prefer not categories of illness but degrees of difficulty – how much of a particular problem behaviour someone displays, rather than which category they fit into. Detailed research work by academic psychologists to relate disorders to the 'big five' personality dimensions (extraversion, neuroticism, agreeableness, conscientiousness and openness to experience) has been undertaken, but – as for the psychiatric attempts to define 'severity' – with little impact on clinical practice.

These different sub-categories of PD are therefore not particularly helpful or insightful by themselves. They describe only clusters of problematic behaviour, and it is only when combined with a psychological or psychodynamic formulation that they provide any meaningful understanding to the service user, or helpful information to guide treatment. A good formulation will describe the 'why' behind the diagnosis, in terms of emotional development, suggested defence mechanisms or cognitive processes.

Good formulation underlies almost any effective psychological treatment for PD, whether we take the psychiatric/diagnostic route or the psychological/dimensions route, but it does not give any indication of where on the spectrum somebody, or indeed oneself, might sit. An explanation that I often give to service users is that all these problems can vary from mild to severe, and from one part of a person's life to another: 'everybody has a personality and nobody is perfect'.

Evolving health service policy on PD

Within mental health services, it is only since 2003 that official Department of Health service policy in the UK came to fully recognise PD as a legitimate condition for statutory services to treat, when the National Institute for Mental Health in England (NIMHE) produced a 'policy implementation guide' (Department of Health/NIMHE, 2003a) insisting that PD should be *'no longer a diagnosis of exclusion'*. This document launched the Department of Health's National PD Development Programme, with three main areas of activity: young people (preventive work), forensic (shared with the Ministry of Justice) and community services, with 11 pilot projects across England, each very different in focus.

The Department of Health and NIMHE also published a sister document for workforce development, *Breaking the Cycle of Rejection: The personality disorder capabilities framework* (2003b). This has since been developed and is now known as the Knowledge and Understanding Framework, with national implementation across all relevant agencies and disciplines starting in 2009.

In 2009, the Department of Health held a presentation in 10 regions of the UK to present and explain its commissioning guidance, *Recognising Complexity* (Department of Health, 2009b). This guidance highlighted that the following in particular contribute to making PD more problematic than other mental health diagnoses:

- a 'whole system' approach is needed
- service user partnership is especially important
- there is a lack of evidence.

Whole system consequences arise because PD is a disturbance of relationships – and many of these relationships are with the statutory services and those who try to offer help. With the hypersensitivities inherent in the condition, this frequently leads to attempts to help being perceived as obstructive, intrusive or frankly abusive unless practitioners are extraordinarily sensitive, or suitably trained. The consequent increase in anxiety and perception of injustice can reverberate throughout various agencies involved with a client, leading to a spiral of increased defensiveness by staff and further disturbance in service users.

As a result, poor co-ordination across agencies has directly harmful effects and any 'splitting' between or within them is likely to increase the problems substantially – and often leads to a chronic situation where nothing gets resolved and formal complaints and grievance processes are escalated to senior managerial staff who have none of the necessary expertise or training to resolve it.

Service user partnership has been a major factor in the national PD programme. People diagnosed with PD have commonly been in asymmetrical relationships where others have abused their power and done horrible things to the sufferer, and they will therefore be exquisitely sensitive to this being repeated in a clinical setting. By working closely with service users and ex-service users, a trusting and optimistic relationship can be established and maintained.

This needs to be reflected in local services if they are to be effective. Where service users feel that they are being 'controlled' or 'told what's good for them' they are likely to feel negative and behave accordingly – either by making treatment very difficult for those trying to give it, or by having no confidence that it will be any help, and therefore not engaging. The solution to this demands a certain 'quality of relationship' between staff and service users that is accepting, open and honest, with an explicit and shared understanding of the boundaries.

There is a lack of evidence, or at least of the conclusively and formally researched evidence required for NICE recommendations. This in part explains why PD is still a condition in an early phase of recognition and development, and this means it is much less understood than most other mental disorders. The difficulties in engagement and the often strong emotional reactions from others, which are so characteristic of PD, have also inhibited both research and better understanding.

Many in the field argue that because it is a complex condition it will require complex interventions (rather than simple 'mono-mode' therapies), which will in turn need complex research (including, for whole system work, involvement from disciplines and agencies not traditionally involved in psychiatric research) to achieve better understanding and services. Even those using only the tools of biomedical academic research acknowledge that it is likely to require the development of new approaches and methodologies.

Determining the severity of PD

Recognising Complexity (Department of Health, 2009b) measures severity by the extent to which each of the following five domains are affected.

1. Diagnosis.
2. Pervasiveness.
3. Risk.
4. Complexity/co-morbid conditions.
5. Manageability.

Services consider these five different variables when determining the degree of difficulty an individual may be having, and use it to assess the need to intervene. Each of these areas is dealt with below.

Diagnosis: both multiplicity (the more of the diagnoses from each of the three clusters mentioned above that seem to apply) and any dimensional score (for example, of the total score on one of the validated instruments such as the IPDE-77 screening questionnaire). It is generally acknowledged by clinicians that the more problem areas for relationships that are diagnosable in an individual, the more severe the condition is – although there is no single way to agree this between different clinicians, researchers, services or organisations.

Pervasiveness: how many different areas of life are affected. Those severely affected by their PD are affected in many areas of their lives: intimate, family and social relationships; occupational and educational activity; self-care; likelihood of self-neglect or self-harm; reckless/risky behaviour and lack of initiative. One measure of severity is the number of these different domains in which there is problematic functional impairment.

Risk: to self or to others. Those severely affected by PD may have very persistent and life-threatening self-harming behaviours, or present a very high suicide or self-neglect risk. Because of the nature of their offending behaviours they may also present a risk to other people.

Complexity: the presence of other problems as well, sometimes called co-morbidity. PD is often associated with a range of other conditions such as a history of substance misuse, eating disorders, self-harm behaviours and suicide, criminal offending, poor child care, poor self-care and many other dysfunctional behaviours. The number or severity of these other problems can be used to indicate the severity of PD.

Manageability: dysfunctional behaviours that are associated with PD will often require more intensive community services or joint National Offender Management Service management, or may make community management problematic. To some extent it may be as much a question of staff training or the design of the service, but otherwise, as a consequence of the degree of severity of the above factors or failure of past treatment, some people cannot be effectively and safely contained even by intensive dedicated services.

PD in healthcare problems

With such high levels of disabling difficulties, one might think that there would be many people admitted to hospital with a diagnosis of PD. In fact, the number of admissions for specific treatment of PD is very small because the fundamental diagnosis is rarely used in a way that is registered for the officially collated figures. The figure cited in *No Longer a Diagnosis of Exclusion* (Department of Health/NIMHE, 2003a) (between 36% and 68% in psychiatric inpatient care) highlights this. The condition is clearly very prevalent in the hospitalised population, but it is not often diagnosed.

UK data on the primary diagnosis stated for inpatient psychiatric admissions by region (ie. for *all* hospitals in the region) between 2002 and 2007, are in single figures for four UK regions, and never over 100 in any one region. If these figures accurately reflect the levels of PD in the population as a whole, this would suggest rates of 0.002 to 0.036 per million of the population.

Yet the extent to which PD may be missed or misread suggests that surveys of the population may be a more reliable guide than official statistics. As suggested earlier, such surveys suggest levels of PD of at least four per cent – and some studies have assessed the levels of PD in the population at large at much higher levels, even in one case up to 14%. As PD is, almost by definition, not simply episodic, but a long-term and debilitating condition, this would suggest that overlooking this issue may mean overlooking a major part of the overall 'burden of ill-health' of the nation.

There are also similarly careful studies, outlined earlier and in Peter Cockersell's paper in Chapter 15, exploring the suggestion that there are the greatest concentrations of PD in particular areas where people with problems tend to go, such as homelessness hostels, accident and emergency departments and prisons. More recently, studies of individuals with clear PD characteristics (though not necessarily diagnosed as such) within several healthcare populations suggest that the problems are indeed widespread, both in GP surgeries, and in the caseload of mental health teams, just as they are in the prison population and in homelessness services.

Numerous reasons for this may be considered, from stigma to custom and practice, to poor staff training, and many others. What these figures fail to highlight is the stark reality of life in most acute psychiatric wards. It would be no exaggeration to say that people with PD are often admitted to inpatient psychiatric wards, but current interpretations of the regulations for running acute psychiatric hospitals and the training of most acute ward staff render them unfit for purpose. There is a serious question here about the extent to which iatrogenic harm (harm caused by the attempted healer) is being done.

For purposes of public health then, there is a striking mismatch. Official health service figures seem to show low 'need', but epidemiology suggests this is a very large public health problem indeed. Small wonder then that one concerned clinician has suggested that *'the health professions are hiding from view one of the major sources of suffering and health service costs'* (Tyrer, 2008).

One reason for this under-recognition may be the feature of complex co-morbidity referred to earlier – especially with addictions or other substance abuse, or, it seems, the high prevalence of PD mixed with mental illness among populations with other stated diagnoses that *are* admitted to mental health care, as the figures for Community Mental Health Teams (CMHTs) and Assertive Outreach (AO) services would suggest. Is it then just that health professionals don't want to use the PD diagnosis, and prefer to confer other, and especially more medical, diagnoses?

Indeed, the recent trend of the popular press to reveal celebrities' diagnosis of 'bipolar' may be part of a similar impetus to take responsibility away from individuals by using medical terminology. Emotional instability is a diagnostic feature of borderline PD as well as its formal ICD name, and over-ready display of emotion is an indicator of the histrionic type. To what extent, for example, is 'rapid mood cycling' in bipolar disorder really a separate entity, with a name that suggests a neurobiological cause, rather than an intelligible if erratic human response to difficult emotions?

Perhaps it would be more intellectually honest to admit that there will probably never be a clear line between such clinical conditions, except in the attitudes and responses generated in others. We could describe the whole spectrum of these disorders as having 'bio-psycho-social' causes, and not assume faulty wiring or faulty chemistry as the primary aetiology until it has been specifically proven – as is probably the case for what was once called 'manic-depressive psychosis'.

It is also important to ask whether the diagnosis helps anyway, when it is so associated with stigma and therapeutic nihilism. In two respects at least, it must do. First, the low 'diagnostic visibility' of PD in healthcare certainly does not mean low need. Rather it seems to mean that these needs are not being recognised and are being misread, and as a consequence mismanaged, within the health service. If so, this may translate into a huge number of unnecessary and inappropriate 'investigations' and treatments for problems whose root cause lies elsewhere.

The second reason, however, is that the under-recognition of PD in the health service seems to be counterbalanced by a much higher prevalence in the prison population and amongst homeless people. This suggests, at the very least, that we must now make far greater efforts to bring together healthcare with prison service and homelessness management.

In the case of the prison service, that connection is at least now well recognised in UK policy priorities. The offender health strategy (Department of Health, 2011b) received government backing in 2011, and has ambitions to significantly improve mental health care practice in all areas of offender management. In relation to the homeless population, that process is only now beginning.

Promoting innovative treatments

For those who fear the old therapeutic nihilism that is associated with the diagnosis, we can at least now assert with confidence that PD can no longer be seen as 'untreatable' – one of the things said for many years. It is simply that the old ways of conventional psychiatric care did not work. The same could be said, however, of almost all psychiatric treatments until at least the middle of the last century, and even now many question the adequacy and efficacy of the treatments we do have.

In 2004, the Department of Health announced a programme of development of more innovative services. Throughout the country 11 community pilot sites were chosen to explore and demonstrate new ways of working with PD. They varied from therapeutic communities to individual therapy clinics, from managed clinical networks to walk-in centres and from early intervention to intensive treatment programmes. They utilised various therapeutic approaches and employed between six and 30 staff of various disciplines, most of whom were in the mental health sector, but some were voluntary or community organisations.

A formal multi-method evaluation study was undertaken by Imperial College London and published by the National Institute of Health Research's Service Delivery Organisation in 2007 (Crawford, 2007). Details of this evaluation, and of the development of further services, can be found in the 'Innovation Centres' section of the national PD website: www.personalitydisorder.org.uk.

As a result of this increasing recognition of PD as a relevant issue, the Department of Health commissioned NICE to prepare guidelines for treatment of borderline PD and antisocial PD. The role of NICE is to pronounce on effective treatments that the UK health service should endorse and fund, and these guidelines were issued in 2009 (NICE, 2009a; 2009b). The headlines state that:

- PD *is* treatable
- an optimistic and trusting relationship is required
- there is little randomised control trial evidence to guide specific treatment
- an 'integrated theoretical approach' is needed
- short-term therapy is generally unhelpful
- medication is generally unhelpful
- care needs to be structured, with varying levels of engagement possible
- training is needed, not just in mental health services, but across all sectors.

Thoughts about engaging with complexity

With the development of the national PD programme, and with the wider development and recognition of new ways of working and thinking of PD, we can hope for many new insights and approaches to emerge. In Section two we will outline some of the insights that we may begin to draw from services working mainly outside the health service. For the moment, let us conclude with just a few thoughts on the lessons from the PD programme pilots themselves.

'Complex needs'

Recognising Complexity, the title of the Department of Health's commissioning guidance, seems apt; these are genuinely complex cases in several ways (Department of Health, 2009b). It has also become the commonest service title adopted for the new PD services, usually with full service user input. 'Services for those with complex needs' is universally more popular than 'personality disorder services'.

This is arguably simply a more sanitised term (it is certainly less pejorative), but importantly it is accurate. People who present for help with PD issues rarely come with a single diagnosis, so pervasive is the presence of PD throughout their lives. Co-morbidity, especially with addictions, increases complexity substantially; triple diagnosis even more so – which probably accounts for the very high levels of PD found by earlier studies in CMHTs and AO teams.

However, we still have to recognise that people with PD will often have no diagnosis at all – not because they do not have the symptoms and difficulties that are required for a PD diagnosis, but simply because the diagnosis has not been made. This is not just 'disguised PD', or a reluctance, inability or failure of clinicians to spot the underlying problems, but recognition of PD is more often dependent on sector and setting. Where diagnosis is not the normal way of identifying cases for intervention, the diagnosis is not needed and does not help, and so there will be less or often no diagnosis going on.

Meanwhile, there are still detractors both within the medical and even within the psychiatric profession. There are still many who will say, 'These diagnoses are so uncertain – and these treatments relatively unproven – so what can we be expected to do? We are mental health services, treatment services. It's not our business.' However, this is becoming increasingly untenable as a justification to continue doing nothing. When we look at the overall cost to the economy and the hidden costs to the health service of failing to find better ways, it is hard to justify turning a blind eye to such levels of distress and damage.

Engagement issues

The particular approach or tradition of therapy adopted is probably not the most important factor in meeting complex needs. More relevant factors are probably whole-system co-ordination and the effective engagement of those who are hard to engage. Issues including autonomy and choice, valuing the fact and the nature of relationships, and working with hope and optimism, seem to be most critical in this area of therapy as, of course, in many others.

If the approach taken is too narrow, too circumscribed by advance planning, or too directive, it will not succeed. Simple flow charts or decision trees usually fail. This is partly because people with lifetime experiences of traumatic rejection can be made to feel hopeless about treatment by very small things. These may be conscious, such as careless wording, hurried gestures or wrong body language, or unconscious and irrational factors that are well out of conscious awareness (of both therapist and service user), causing disruptive emotions and a rupture of the therapeutic alliance. These are often not amenable to logic or reason.

Services have to be adept at managing uncertainty and turbulence – things don't go to plan. However, this is part and parcel of the need for positive engagement, not passivity, in treatment. Service models must allow for all the participants to feel that they are being listened to, and they must be given a sense of personal choice – or human agency. Needless to say, this is easier said than done, and is not a simple requirement to put on a service specification. The recent work on enabling environments (EEs), psychologically informed planned environments (PIPEs) and psychologically informed environments (PIEs) goes some way towards defining this. A brief account follows, although more detail is given in Section three of this book.

Enabling environments

The work we started a few years ago at the Royal College of Psychiatrists' Centre for Quality Improvement was to distil the 'essential ingredients' from the Community of Communities standards, based on work we did about their underlying values, and produce a list of 10 attributes of an environment that demonstrated that it was 'psychologically healthy' – an 'enabling environment'. It could apply as much to an office or classroom as to a prison wing or hospital unit. These 10 qualities have now been piloted and can be used as a hallmark of quality, with an award that organisations get by submitting a satisfactory portfolio of evidence (which might be photos or artwork, just as much as official documents) and having a confirmation visit. The pilots have been very successful and will soon be launched on the world, and anybody who wants to is invited to apply for the award and be taken through the process.

Psychologically informed planned environments

A PIPE can be seen as a specially structured and defined EE developed in and for the criminal justice sector, which has been through the policy grinder and come out the other side in a form that is recognisable to 'those who matter' in the civil service hierarchy. However, a different way of looking at it would be to describe a PIPE as something between an EE (which is about recognising very general qualities of an environment) and a therapeutic community (which is a highly structured and accredited programme). Nonetheless, the preparation work on developing PIPEs is well underway. The first pilot PIPEs were set up in 2011, and training for staff (including KUF) is an important ingredient in this.

Psychologically informed environments

These are PIPEs with the 'pee' taken out of them, if you like, so they do not need the level of advance planning and prior approval that PIPEs must have. They may arise spontaneously, and will often be developed by less formal processes (Johnson & Haigh, 2010).

The main focus of encouragement to PIEs is currently coming from the Department for Communities and Local Government (CLG), which is responsible for housing and homelessness policy. PIEs in homelessness services therefore concentrate on improving provision such as hostels and refuges for homeless people – and they are starting by identifying and showcasing existing good practice. A very helpful guidance paper, has been published on the CLG's website (CLG/NMHDU, 2010) and further guidance is promised. Policy makers, commissioners and providers in the homeless and housing sector all seem to be confident that this is a good and cost-effective answer to a problem that cannot be legislated away.

In all of these models, the efforts and training of individual staff need to be supported, expressed and carried through into the work and the 'feel' of the service as a whole. Otherwise their efforts will be undermined, running counter to other subtler messages of rejection, to which this client group will be especially sensitive. Considerations must include the atmosphere, the daily routines, the care pathways, the rules, even the colour schemes, lighting and furnishings. We need environments that feel 'safe' – not too municipal, corporate or institutional – places where people with dispossessed lives can go, feel accepted, talk, or just 'be'.

Summary

The concept of PD, though a deeply problematic diagnosis and a highly stigmatising label, is nevertheless now offering a useful psychological and practical framework for understanding and recognising statutory provision needs for those in unsatisfactory mental health services, or prison, or those who are homeless.

This needs to be done:

- without interdisciplinary or cross-agency rivalries, so the whole system is not split into competing interests
- through full partnership with service users and ex-service users, so a sense of ownership is generated, and a sense of belonging is developed
- with continual attention to the quality of relationships, and a willingness to examine and improve them.

Editor's comment: The science behind psychiatry

We can see the new insights that can be drawn from a combination of in-depth clinicians' understanding of the phenomenon of PD, with the survey-led perspective that results from a more epidemiological approach.

It is now time to look in more detail at the science of the nature of trauma – the natural history of trauma. For this, however, we will need a very broad overview, covering a wide canvas of different disciplines and knowledge bases. We must consider not just contemporary biology and neuroscience, but also psychology and other areas of social science, and the actual practice of frontline services and other agencies in civil society.

These will then lead us to rediscover the need to bring together research science with actual practice in order to gain a fuller understanding of human experience.

Chapter 2
Perspectives from the biological sciences

Robin Johnson

'The brain continually changes to reflect aspects of its environment. In other words, its neural architecture comes to reflect the environment that shapes it...' (Lou Cozolino, 2002)

Introduction

Only 20 years ago, it was not implausible to believe that the mapping of the human genome would soon reveal the underlying blueprint of our lives, our fundamental characteristics as a species and even our individual personalities. We heard talk of 'the gene', not merely for cancer or Huntington's, but also for schizophrenia, for depression, and of course 'the gay gene'. So widespread and contagious was the optimism with which this hope was pursued, that some of the vocabulary escaped into popular culture. It is now common to hear people say that this or that belief or loyalty or behaviour 'is in our DNA' – meaning it's part of what makes us who we are.

However, with the mapping of the genome completed, this hope for a single, authoritative 'source code' answer to 'why we are as we are' became untenable. We now know that there are some 20–25,000 genes in the human genome, but the human body is composed of between 50 and 70 trillion individual cells. There are some 30 billion neurons in the cortex of the human brain alone, and potentially a million billion synaptic connections between neurons. There are simply far too few genes for there to be any one-to-one correlation between one gene and one characteristic – let alone for highly complex behaviour.

To some extent, the yearning to find the science that explains why we are as we are has not gone, but moved on to find a new home, and the most likely source of new insights into the human condition within the 'hard' sciences now seems to lie not in the genome, but in the close study of the architecture and functioning of our brains – in neuroscience. With the added attraction of new technologies – fMRI, EEG, PET and CAT scans etc – creating eye-catching imagery that looks good on the page or screen, we now seek to find the ultimate explanation of our natures in how we – that is, our brains – are 'hard-wired' for a, b, or c.

Yet if it is now impossible to argue that broad behavioural characteristics can be predetermined in any detail by the genes that generate the brain, it is also untenable that specific neural connections can likewise control behaviour. Instead we must see these and many other features as essentially developmental. That is, they arise in a complex process of interaction between the gene pool and the environment. It is this that leaves many of our key characteristics open, to some extent, to variation in the developing process.

The full significance of this in terms of the nature of the brain is still emerging, but one aspect of this phenomenon, which goes by the name of neural plasticity, is now becoming clear. The significance of plasticity for the human susceptibility to trauma is central to our developing understanding of the natural history of trauma: the causes, the natural course, and also the things that we can do to intervene.

The developing infant brain

There is an extensive body of well-evidenced science to show that the body responds to the experience of anxiety by a release of chemical messengers, whose task is to prepare the body for fight or flight, mobilising us for action. There is now good reason to believe that prolonged stress – stress without the immediate release that fight or flight brings – leads to a build-up of the residue of these chemical triggers in the system.

Prolonged build-up may then compromise, among other things, the auto-immune system, which is put on hold for the fight-flight reaction, so that over time our resistance to diseases is impaired. It has been shown, for example, that the body under psychological stress mends more slowly even from a simple flesh wound (Glaser & Kiecolt-Glaser, 1994), and it has recently been argued that long-term stress may be the link between unsatisfactory life circumstances and eventual depression (Foresight, 2008).

Some recent neuroscience now suggests that the experience of neglect or outright abuse in infancy or childhood can equally affect the development of the brain of the infant. We can easily imagine how, before birth, the biochemistry of maternal distress – a chemical wash of regulatory hormonal or endocrinal systems – might be passed on to the child in the womb (summarised in Wilkinson, 2006; DiPietro *et al*, 2010).

However, the same build-up of the biochemistry of stress, it is argued, can be passed on to the infant after birth. When the biochemistry of stress is a constant phenomenon, this produces constantly high levels of these chemical triggers in the developing infant brain. This can then lead – especially perhaps during critical or 'sensitive' developmental stages in infancy – to anomalous brain development in the infant, in the form of reduced density of neural growth in key areas (Perry *et al*, 1995; Perry, 2005; Teicher *et al*, 2003; Galderisi & Mucci, 2000).

This may make for the establishment of a pattern of neural stimulations with an *'electrochemical baseline'*, which is chronically *'blunted by habituation to risk'* (James, 2008). Moreover, these emotional/chemical influences have their impact, just as the infant brain is developing and finding its way in the world, in just those areas of brain architecture (the amygdala, the limbic system etc) that are now thought to be implicated in complex social and cognitive functions in adults, such as emotional regulation, 'affiliative behaviour', attachment bonding and empathy (Benjamin *et al,* 2009).

Psychologists indicate that it is underlying difficulties in exactly these areas that are then associated with behavioural problems. This possible causal chain would then seem to provide both the physiological and psychological underpinning for difficulties in later life such as compulsive risk-seeking behaviour, impulsivity, aggression, emotional volatility and/or a failure to respond to cues that indicate that a particular behaviour or emotion may be dysfunctional in context.

These are precisely the behaviours that, in extreme cases, would lead to the individual in question being diagnosed with a personality disorder (PD). The link between trauma and PD seems, therefore, to be lodged into the brain at a very early stage. The neuroscience of childhood trauma literature naturally raises concerns that the developmental impact of stress and trauma in childhood may be irreversible, or if not entirely irreversible then at least markedly less responsive or amenable to change via later influences and experiences.

If we are right to infer that these difficulties in later life would lead to the individual being given a diagnosis of PD, then these studies of the developing brain would seem to echo and perhaps confirm earlier concerns that PD is essentially not treatable. The most that we should be able to hope for, on this account, is to be able to mitigate or at least to contain the consequences of such inner vulnerability in later life.

One reason for caution in this argument, however, is the fact that these suggestions of the likely long-term impact of childhood trauma are predicting a future that we have not yet seen. There are as yet few if any studies to assess the actual later fate of children who had been both subjected to stress, and then laboratory tested for certitude as to the accuracy of the associations found. Such studies would be hard to construct, expensive to conduct, and in order to meet the rigorous standards of medicine (Goldacre, 2008), great care would be needed to ensure that full randomised control trial standards are met.

A further reason for caution lies in the wide disparity between the precision tools we have for identifying these apparent biomarkers, and those we have for the consequences. The high degree of specificity in the language of biology – cortisol, limbic system, anterior cingulate cortex etc – and the relatively fine grain of the technology that allows us to view neural structures and activity so intimately is simply not matched by any comparable clarity of tools, or even of basic concepts, for the suggested emotional and social consequences (Dingwall, 1989; Dingwall *et al,* 2003).

As we have already seen in Chapter 1, even the basic medical vocabulary of diagnosis is fairly unreliable here, and all other categories of adverse outcome, as seen, managed and counted by other agencies, are inevitably offering complex accounts of multi-faceted and multi-factorial problems (Fahmy, 2009) and to some extent circumstantial evidence. Even when we can trace – without interfering with – the natural life courses of children believed to be at risk, the evidence of difficult, conflict-ridden and messy lives is likely to be difficult, conflict-ridden and messy evidence.

Finally, the neuroscience of childhood trauma raises very serious concerns and has prompted calls for early intervention, from clinicians and politicians alike (Allen & Duncan Smith, 2010). The precise nature and focus of this remedial intervention is less clear, however, and not easily derived from the neuroscience itself. What may work, to intervene, will have to be an exploratory and empirical process, proven by its successes only many years later, just as it always has been.

Corroboration from animal studies

There is some further evidence that might be taken to corroborate the prediction that early trauma can lead to behavioural problems in later life, and it comes from the science of ethology – the study of animals' behaviour, not solely in laboratory conditions but in their natural context. It is particularly significant for these new interpretations that recent studies of other mammals provide corroborating evidence that these developmental mechanisms, and the vulnerability they allow, are deeply rooted in biology.

In the 1950s, in a long series of laboratory studies of monkeys, the psychologist Harlow and his colleagues (Suomi & Harlow, 1971) were able to gain some remarkable insights on the importance of affection and play in the healthy growth of monkey young – including some highly poignant observations of baby monkeys craving comfort and of under-comforted monkeys growing into emotionally stunted adults, unable to nurture their own young. (These studies and their significance are briefly reviewed in Chapter 5.)

There are also now many studies of rats that show that in an 'enriched environment' – by which we mean a cage with a number of things that they will find stimulating (Greenfield, 2000) – rats will show a very healthy growth of neural connections, while in other studies, the biochemistry of stress that we find in humans is replicated in rats (Wilkinson, 2006). These studies allow us to confirm in consistent and controlled laboratory conditions that maternal care in other mammals, for example, has a discernible material (ie. biological) impact on the young, with lasting effects on future behaviour.

However, it is the growing number of studies of animals in their natural environments, and especially of primates (with whom we share most of our DNA and much of our essential brain architecture (Williamson & Allman, 2011)), that now reveals still more relevant observations. For example, baboons will respond to stress, and to changes of status in the hierarchy of the troop with much the same biochemical markers that we humans use (Sapolsky, 1998).

Taken together, these studies seem to strongly suggest that stress and the phenomenon of early adaptation is biological in essence – that is, they would at least indicate that these mechanisms precede the development of any of the more sophisticated psychological elements that are characteristic of humans and our social world.

Psychological damage or evolutionary adaptation?

So far back do these patterns of development go in the various species of primates of which we humans are, after all, only one branch, that it has been suggested that there may be something quite fundamental in the evolutionary advantage given by the inheritance of a wide range of development processes. The adaptability that is then conferred upon a species will increase the variability in the population of any species, in response to differing environments (Wilkinson, 2006; Wilkinson & Pickett, 2009; Howarth, 2009), without reliance solely on the inherently more risky random mutation of genes.

The ultimate explanation for the inheritance of adaptability may lie deep within the Darwinian framework, without which it is often said nothing in biology makes sense (Rose, 2006). This line of argument is central to one of the newer and more exciting areas of biology that are now stepping in as the hopes for the human genome as the ultimate explanation start to recede. This new area of scientific analysis goes by the name of epigenetics (Carey, 2011; Burkeman, 2010).

At its core is the suggestion that later events in the course of development of the embryo will influence the 'expression' of the genome – the turning on and off of particular genes, in sequence – so that development processes, rather than simply following automatically from the original endowment of DNA, are in fact highly responsive to the environment.

A worker bee, a drone and a queen, are genetically identical, yet their adult physical form and their behaviour, though programmed entirely by the same genes, are radically different. A small oak might become a towering tree, or a bonsai miniature, according to circumstances (Bateson & Gluckman, 2011; for further examples, see Cohen & Stewart, 1994).

This phenomenon also applies to humans. There is now growing evidence, for example, that poor nutrition in childhood leads to a physiological development that is optimally attuned to a world of poor nutrition, but not well attuned to conditions of plenty. As we have seen, nutrients are not the only influential aspect of the chemical wash in which the young human grows that will have an impact on the development of the embryo and infant during these formative stages. The umbilical cord carries information in the form of stress hormones on the state of the environment in which the child will grow up – and for which the embryonic child is then prepared (Wilkinson & Pickett, 2009; DiPietro *et al*, 2010).

These developmental mechanisms for adapting to the environment appear then to be an entirely natural phenomenon, rather than an illness, with their origins, in evolutionary terms, in providing a protective element against what appear to be likely adverse conditions in the world the embryo child is being born to, or the infant growing up in. Even in the womb, it seems, when the going gets tough, the tough get going.

This interpretation marks a significant step beyond earlier accounts of evolutionary psychology (Ardrey, 1961; Morris, 1966; Alland, 1967; Wilson, 1975; Tooby & Cosmides, 1992; Pinker, 1997), which had argued that our basic psychological processes, characteristics and behaviour were fixed at a genetic level by the dictates of survival as a species on the open savannah plains of Africa, where the first of the genus *Homo* first made their appearance.

Certainly there is a very real genetic component to all this. Part of the excitement of the 'epigenetic revolution' – and one of the reasons it might justify such a name (Carey, 2011; Burkeman, 2010) – is that it suggests that the old debates over the respective roles of nature and nurture have finally had their day. It is not so much that we are a mixture of nature and nurture, but that it really no longer seems tenable to suggest that they are two different things (Cohen & Stewart, 1994; Ridley, 2003; O'Shea, 2005; Rose, 2005; Bateson & Gluckman, 2011); there simply is no real difference, no such division in biological reality.

It now seems that the role of our genetic inheritance is to provide variability, not fixity. What is more, that variability continues to develop long after birth, and most markedly so in us humans, as new experiences finally take over from genes as the main source of environmental stimulus and ongoing responsive development, through learning. The key discovery here is the recognition, emerging through the latter half of the 20th century, of the phenomenon of neural plasticity.

Neural plasticity and the pliable brain

'Plasticity' here means malleability – the capacity to take different shapes – and things that are plastic may be moulded and then harden into a particular given form.

The plasticity of the brain operates at many levels, from the macroscopic (flexible features of brain architecture) to the microscopic (the signalling of neurons and the connectivity between them, at scales of micro-millimetres). Thus the term neural plasticity covers a number of related phenomena, but all have in common the central fact that brain circuitry wires in response to lived experience, and some brain circuitry, at least, may constantly re-wire.

It has been known for some time that particular areas of the brain appear to specialise in particular functions, such as speech, motor control or balance. Some thinkers have gone so far as to suggest that the brain is therefore constructed rather like a Swiss Army knife, with many different specialist functions, and that they do not necessarily work well together as a whole. Do we have here some quite fundamental design flaws, and might this then partly explain why we as humans seem to have so many consistent weaknesses in our thinking and reactions (Marcus, 2008)? If so, then even a slight developmental impairment in any one area, upsetting the precarious whole, might help explain the particularly flawed performance of some individuals and be partly to blame for the volatile chemistry and volatile behaviour of those who have severe emotional and social problems.

However, the extent to which these 'early parts of our brains' have refused to evolve further has since been debated (Butler & Hodos, 2005; Patton, 2008); and now there is in any case growing evidence (Doidge, 2007) that the degree of 'localisation' of functions in the brain may also have been overstated. The brain has evolved to work as a whole, and while normally entrusting certain functions to certain areas, it does so more pragmatically, and can, when necessary, 'recruit' spare capacity in one area when extra learning power is needed in a different field (Doidge, 2007; Levitin, 2007).

We are familiar with the idea that blind people may have especially acute hearing and that those who learn Braille can develop an acuity of sense through their fingertips that most of us do not have. However, more recent developments suggest that the blind can also learn to 'see' by learning to read the signals from images projected onto the skin of the back. More remarkable still, other studies now suggest that recovery from major neurological damage, such as from a stroke, is also achievable, as the brain gradually finds ways to bring into use other undamaged areas, co-opted to serve the functions of the areas that have been disabled. This can be a permanent re-wiring to cope with new demands, but it may also be a temporary borrowing. Moreover, this phenomenon goes very deep.

If the brain can re-wire even its major structural features in response to a need in order to compensate for a deficiency, then the question must arise as to whether the brain also provides us with similar multiple mechanisms to restore useful functional flexibility after early maladaptation. We might then especially expect to find this restorative capacity in the area of learned behaviour, which is the aspect of existence most susceptible to variation in repertoire. This is how we are most open to new formative experience. And given the right support, we can learn new ways.

These discoveries of the flexible architecture of the brain are remarkable, but they are in fact only two further examples in human neurology of a much more pervasive phenomenon found in biology, for which the neurologist C H Waddington coined the term homeorhesis (or 'same flow') (Cohen & Stewart, 1994) for the tendency in nature to make available many corrective mechanisms to bring development back on track. In humans – and in many other creatures – the most sophisticated mechanisms for adjusting are through learning from experience.

The evolutionary advantage in learning for enhanced variability

When something happens to us, our brains respond. In the course of experience – including the experience of our own actions, feelings, thoughts and even intentions – new neural connections are made in the brain, and strengthened by repetition. In this way we learn. In and by the physical nature of our brains, via their innate plasticity, actual lived experience is translated into physical changes in the neural connectivity of the brain.

In a sense this should be unsurprising. If it is true – as we have no good reason to doubt (Bennett & Hacker, 2003; Dennett, 2003; Searle, 2007) – that for every lived experience there must be a counterpart in the brain, a 'neural correlate', then the brain must be responding physically to experience.

It is important to remember that this is just the first – though incontrovertible – real evidence that experience is not necessarily secondary to biology, but rather that experience itself causes physical changes in the brain. We now have solid scientific proof, not just of the fact or the logic, but of the actual mechanisms by which life experiences contribute to making us what we are. What is true of biochemical influences in the womb and after remains equally true of actual lived experiences, as children and as adults.

The role of reinforcement

The constant responsiveness of neural plasticity is matched and underpinned by a propensity to strengthen connections that are frequently used – as it is said, the neurons that fire together, wire together (Hebb, 1949). Over time, networks of neurons gradually organise themselves into established pathways (Edelmann, 1992). In this way we learn, and in this way, too, previous experience comes to colour or shape our new experiences, with associations from the past.

In this way our early experience – or any very powerful experience later in life – will be formative. This is expressed and illustrated neatly by Folensbee (2007):

'Current experiences that are similar to old experiences will trigger the old patterns to fire, and these old patterns are likely to influence the brain's processing of the new situation ... If a person has experienced repeated painful personal betrayals throughout childhood, then the slightest hint of disregard displayed by the current spouse will trigger strong emotions related to fear of betrayal that lead to the person misinterpreting the current spouse as being ready to leave – even though the reality is that the current spouse is simply being somewhat pre-occupied.'

We are, it seems, initially hard-wired for very little; we are originally soft-wired and ready for anything. It is our life experience that leads to any particular networks forming and firming up. We are born with on average some 100 billion neurons, and in the first year of life these continue to multiply in sheer number. After that, our brains continue to grow at an amazing rate – doubling in size in our first two years, and increasing by 400% by the time we reach 16 years – not through addition of new neurons, but by the growth of connectivity between them.

In the economy of the brain, it is a case of the survival of the busiest. After the first burst of neuron growth in childhood, then begins a major process of dying off, pruning back and shedding unused or little used neurons and their connections. The most used neurons and their rapidly proliferating connections remain, however, and continue to make new, richer and subtler connections with each other. This associative process is actually accentuated by the process of pruning of the less used neurons. In this way, rather than being 'hard-wired', the more evolutionarily advanced parts of our brains are built to be 'sculpted' by our actual lived experience.

It is only with constant repetition of associations at a neurological level that the connectivity between nerve cells and networks gradually firms up, and yet there remain plenty more connections only loosely wired to others, able to fire and respond to any new situation in a new way; the malleability remains, as without it we could not deal with new experiences.

Reinforcement and trauma

It is not clear to what extent this constancy of repetition is also necessary for the maintenance and strengthening of synaptic connections related to traumatic experience. Ethical considerations mean that we cannot submit research subjects to overwhelmingly traumatising stress, and then see if their brain scanning shows re-sculpting comparable to that from long-term exposure. It is likely in principle that any very powerfully charged experience – including very positive experience – may in itself create stronger associations.

However, it is consistent with what we do know to suggest that it is the constant reprocessing of traumatising experience in thought and memory that may provide the cyclical reinforcement that entrenches the neural pathways. The question that this raises is whether ongoing life experiences recreate the scenarios that re-enact, reconfirm and embed earlier traumatised pathways, or whether they free us from them?

The mounting body of evidence for the lasting impact of trauma at sensitive periods in infancy is now counterbalanced by these other strands in contemporary neuroscience, which allow hugely more scope in principle for adaptive learning throughout life, and thus for recovery. The suggestion that early maladaptation necessarily predicts later life appears to be premature. That, at least, is the case for optimism, but we must also bear in mind that learning can mean learning further maladaptive responses too.

As we have seen, the neurons that survive the first pruning in childhood and a second major wave again in adolescence are the ones that are most used, and built upon, in later life. Subsequently, the inter-neural connections that have most 'traffic' are strengthened to carry still more. In this way, our thought patterns do influence our reactions to events; and they form part of the cluster of behaviours, perceptions and emotions – what psychologists call our 'schemas' – with which we deal with new experiences. The world then responds, in turn, to our behaviour, and so the cycles continue.

Plasticity and self-fulfilling prophesy

In this way, then, repeated experience in later life could play a large role in the maintenance of our customary thought patterns. If we continue to generate the same behaviour, relationships and experiences, the same circuitry will again fire, and the same neural connections will be strengthened. We then have a self-organising, self-maintaining cycle (Cohen & Stewart, 1994; Capra, 1997; Rose, 2006).

This opens a whole new avenue of enquiry as to why we may find unwanted repetitive patterns in behaviour. If the continuing impact of early traumas and schemas works through cycles of behaviour and experience that can be interrupted, then at least in principle it may be possible to intercept such patterns of repetition and reinforcement if managed with care.

It now seems, therefore, that the ability to change and to respond to new experiences is deeply rooted in us, biologically and neurologically. However, this then raises questions about fixed behaviours in a world that is constantly changing and full of new experiences. Why and how does plasticity seem to open up new life opportunities for some, but not for others? And most importantly, why do some people who have had experiences of abuse, neglect or trauma in childhood find themselves stuck in patterns of self-defeating behaviour?

Two alternative hypotheses arise:

- Full neurological embedding of trauma, and its long aftermath, may depend on how strong, deep, or early the formative traumatising experiences were.
- Embedding may depend on how constant the repetition of experiences is, reconfirming and entrenching the neural pathways in some cases but not in others.

At this point we might be content to return to the original neuroscience of childhood thesis: that it is early trauma that, at a biological and neurological level, impairs and restricts an individual's repertoire of ways to interact with others. Before we can be confident of this answer, however, we will also need to look further and explore the possible influences of trauma later in life, which may also account for the persistence of repetitive patterns. This we will do, in terms of theoretical perspectives, in the final chapters of this section, and in Section two we will explore these in more depth with examples in actual practice.

Neuroscience findings and diagnostic approaches

Before we do, let us briefly re-visit one last aspect of the neuroscience of trauma, as an example of the kind of questions we now need to ask.

As we have seen, the observations of neuroscience seem to confirm the validity of many of the working concepts that psychology has developed over the course of the 20th century. We should note, however, that these scientifically confirmed psychological concepts do not appear to fit with any great precision, or conform closely to, the formal medical diagnostic categories of PD. There is little so far in these underlying brain-area issues that can be translated readily into an understanding of specific syndromes, such as the supposed antisocial or borderline, schizotypal or paranoid personality types. There would appear to be several possible interpretations for this difference.

The first is that these clinical and diagnostic patterns are simply not supported by evidence from the harder sciences, and therefore they may simply be wrong – or at least misleading and unhelpful, actually contributing to the obscuring of the underlying issues. Making imprecise and arbitrary distinctions via diagnosis may have served to accommodate PD somewhat uneasily within the traditions of medicine, which seem to require detailed formulation and diagnostic precision. However, these apparently precise clusters of symptoms are simply superimposed upon chaotic and fluid experiences that do not lend themselves to such distinctions.

Another possible interpretation is that it is premature to dismiss the possible connections between diagnostic categories of PD and discoveries in neuroscience. The full recognition of the nature and extent of PD is still emerging, and there has not been sufficient time to study the behavioural features that may reflect underlying neuroscientific understandings. For many years, such was the stigma attached to the diagnosis of PD that it was common for an alternative diagnosis to be given when individuals were accepted into mental health services. Now that psychiatry has agreed that PD is not a 'diagnosis of exclusion', the more accurate diagnosis can in principle be given.

Meanwhile, the progress of neuroscience has been so rapid that it is too soon to write off any area of possible implications. Neuro-anatomy is showing us promising new areas for enquiry (Kandel, 1998; LeDoux, 2002;

Williamson & Allman, 2011) and an understanding of plasticity is allowing a new appreciation of the mechanism of therapeutic exchange in psychotherapy (Cozolino, 2002; Doidge, 2007; Fonagy, 2004; Folensbee, 2007) that can encompass PD alongside other forms of distress.

It may be, for example, that these clinically found patterns, the diagnosis of PD and its various sub-types, are in fact reasonably valid, at least in terms of the problems that medicine tends to see in medical caseloads. However, if so, there would appear to be some other, or further, processes of selection or moulding of the presentations and behaviours that medical services have identified. This interpretation would suggest that some other aspects of social process have an additional shaping influence on the phenomena seen in the clinical setting.

We may need a better understanding of how medicine in practice works, through referral mechanisms, assessment and screening systems, and the expectations of co-operation and engagement with treatment that standard psychotherapeutic approaches demand, in order to appreciate why certain problems come to the attention of psychiatry, and so attract a diagnosis. These processes may influence the filtering of cases into the categories that medicine then attempts to identify.

So, for example, we can see that the individual with a borderline PD will seek help when distressed, and their problems will be seen and diagnosed. With some public concern over highly publicised cases of antisocial personalities, we can see how medicine has been asked to explore how psychiatry and psychology may be able to help where the criminal justice system is floundering.

In private sector psychotherapy and analysis, which is more accepted and integrated into the medical profession in the US where the authoritative Diagnostic and Statistical Manuals are produced, those patients who prove hardest to treat may lead the analyst to consider underlying problems such as histrionic or narcissistic tendencies, or similar features, to explain what seems to stand in the way of forming a productive therapeutic relationship.

Perhaps, then, we need to consider more closely how it is that some disruptive behaviour is seen by mental health services, and codified in psychiatry, whereas other behaviour in essentially the same spectrum of distress and damage is seen instead by other professions. This will mean that, to make sense of these patterns, we must look more closely at the way that problems are dealt with in society, by society and its various agencies.

Editor's comment:
Widening the question

Here, we will need to change disciplines, to move from pure biology to social science, and start to draw upon the many studies from social psychology and sociology that examine social processes in adult life. Here we will find many studies that indicate the role of repetitive re-enactment and cyclical reinforcement in day-to-day social interactions.

Such observations will, however, take the epigenetic revolution into wholly new territory, not merely extending beyond the earlier accounts, but entering the sphere previously thought to belong to the fuzzier world of the social sciences. Studies of rats and apes can take us only part of the way. We must now enter the unique and multi-faceted social sphere that humans have elaborated for ourselves, and enter the still newer worlds of neuro-psychoanalysis, neuro-anthropolgy and social neuroscience.

Chapter 3

Perspectives from the social sciences

Robin Johnson

'The available data, though limited, supports the theory that neuronal growth and enhanced interconnection among neurons … parallel the experiential and symptomatic changes we witness in psychotherapy.'
(Lou Cozolino, 2002)

Introduction

Medicine, as the origin of the healing arts, has its roots in understanding illness and finding effective treatments, and so has amassed a working vocabulary of types of illness, diagnosis of symptoms and formal categorisation by disease entities. By contrast, psychology, as a branch of science, has its roots in experiment and statistical analysis rather than in referral clusters for its main subject matter and explanatory frameworks. Psychology, with its origins in the study of normal human behaviour, focuses on such processes as cognition, learning and social function, which are common to all humankind, rather than on the diagnosis of pathology of the few.

In practice, of course, there has been a constant dialogue and exchange between psychiatry and clinical psychology in particular, but the difference in their origins and cultural roots serves to illuminate some differences in their current contributions. For example, the models of human distress and dysfunction that have developed within clinical psychology have consistently tended to identify personal difficulties as a matter of degree, as parts of a continuum, rather than as essentially different entities.

For this reason, arguably, it has been psychology rather than medicine that has tended to develop the concepts of underlying themes and conflicts that have proved more helpful in identifying the key issues in the treatment of personality disorder (PD), as Rex Haigh indicates in Chapter 1.

However, there are other key differences. Medicine is rooted in biology and bodily functions, and here the individual and his environment, and other people, are clearly distinct. But psychology has had no need to start from any separation of individual and social influences in the study of behaviour. Studies in social psychology are part of the bread and butter of psychology, and the responses of other people to our own behaviour and our responses to theirs are a core part of the subject matter of both psychology and sociology, and indeed they form the bridge between them.

Nevertheless, the line between psychology and sociology is sometimes hard to draw. Each has its focus in areas where the other discipline will not normally go; but the overlap between them is in precisely the areas we need to consider next.

Psychology's general focus on the processes of learning, rewards and group processes provides plentiful solid experimental evidence of the importance of feedback of all kinds in reconfirming patterns of experience and of behaviour. There are many studies from experimental social psychology that have explored this territory, aiming to pinpoint the function of cyclical, repetitive re-enactment in learning, and the central role of social reinforcement of behaviour and perceptions. These studies, typically conducted with adults, indicate a multiplicity of ways for later experience to mould future behaviour.

Although the human social world has many areas in which behavioural patterns can seem appropriate or inappropriate, the powerful role of social forces to manage and control our behaviour is a constant. Where individuals' behaviour may differ and respond to a variety of highly idiosyncratic influences, in social and group pressures we see a constant tendency to bring individual experience and behaviour back into the range of the norm. Though some may see this as a form of oppression of the individual – and indeed, it can be – it is a part of how we are made (Gazzaniga, 2009).

However, whereas psychology rests upon a firm grounding in experiment, other areas of social science such as sociology and anthropology, which consider the behaviour of humans in groups, in organisations and in whole cultures, do not have the opportunity to conduct experiments to the same degree. These disciplines are therefore largely reliant on observation and attempts at accurate description married with rigorously systematic interpretation of what is observed.

The link between psychology and neuroscience

Psychology in particular has developed a number of key concepts for features of the human psychological repertoire, both cognitive and emotional, and these now seem to correlate quite closely either to particular aspects of brain anatomy, or to hormonal activity that can now be observed in the brain. Underlying issues of emotional self-regulation, impulsivity or risk taking, impaired attachment, empathy or affiliation, which neuroscience now identifies as key areas of potential difficulty, largely reflect the language and interpretative frameworks of psychology and its healing wing, psychotherapy.

Of these, perhaps the most significant is the neuro-anatomy and biochemistry that underpins what is now commonly known as the attachment system. The pioneering work of John Bowlby (1973; 1980) first drew attention to the importance of attachment behaviour for the dependent infant and explored the problematic consequences in later life if attachment bonds were not securely made in infancy. A central tenet of attachment theory is that early experiences and attachment during infancy then provide a model or foundation for relationships in later life (Zeanah & Shah, 2005).

Bowlby trained as a psychoanalyst, but with a difference: he believed that any interpretations of human emotions needed to be founded in empirical observation derived not only from the consulting rooms, but from human biology and the growing body of animal studies. This approach has produced a great many useful insights into the nature and variety of the emotional difficulties that may result when secure attachments with care givers are not made, or disrupted by, for example, neglect or outright abuse.

Bowlby's theories and clinical observations, soon to be strongly backed by experimental evidence (Ainsworth *et al*, 1978), were highly influential in developing our understanding of the crucial importance of parental care. Allan Schore, one of the first to argue the close corroboration between attachment theory and neuroscience, has argued that *'attachment theory has spawned one of the broadest, most profound and creative lines of research in twentieth century psychology'* because it is a theoretical model that can *'shift back and forth between the psychological and biological levels'* (Carroll, 2000).

Bowlby's work was among the first psychodynamic thinking to be widely accepted within the mainstream science community, in contrast to that of

Freud and many of his immediate successors, whose exclusively clinical practice-based theories and observations lacked the underpinning in more rigorous and empirical biology that has given attachment theory its credence.

So central is this new thinking to our developing understanding of how to work with the aftermath of traumatic experience, that the prospect of re-establishing psychotherapeutic thinking and practice with a firm anchoring now in the 'hard sciences' has rejuvenated the confidence of the advocates of 'talking therapies' of all kinds. Much of this development depends upon the opportunity to re-conceptualise personal change in terms of learning and neural connectivity, and with the emotional or 'affective' aspects of learning now firmly connected to the more conceptual (or 'cognitive') (LeDoux, 1998; 2002; Schore, 1994; Panksepp, 1998; Damasio, 2004; Shotter, 1993; Cromby, 2005). However, the general principle, that learning is enabled and enhanced by biochemical activity in the brain, is now well evidenced (O'Shea, 2005; Rose, 2005).

Moreover, we can see that learning is especially pronounced during sensitive developmental stages, typically in childhood, but is a constantly possible phenomenon throughout life, and the biochemistry that supports neural growth (ie. neural connectivity and thus learning) is rekindled in situations of mild to moderate stress. Once again – and typical of the approach that Bowlby began – it is evolutionary advantage that is seen as the explanatory framework, but now with observations of the brain in action adding to observations from the clinic and the field.

Psychotherapy, enriched environments and neural growth

The concept that neural growth is stimulated by mild to moderate stress was also discussed by Lou Cozolino, American professor of psychology and psychotherapist, in *The Neuroscience of Psychotherapy* (2002), one of the most thoroughly detailed attempts to translate neuroscience's discoveries into psychotherapeutic concepts – and vice versa. Observing that studies show that rats raised in 'enriched environments' (environments with plenty of stimuli) have both more neurons and more synaptic connections between neurons, Cozolino notes that:

'During periods of stress, changes in the bio-chemical environment of the brain shifts its focus to new learning. Although extreme stress inhibits new learning, mild to moderate stress stimulates neural growth hormones and

leads to increased production of cells in brain areas involved in learning … Stressful and dangerous situations alert and prepare the brain to pay attention and learn…' (pp23–24)

Cozolino therefore suggests that psychotherapy should be considered as the human equivalent of such an enriched environment, similarly promoting the development of cognitive, emotional and behavioural abilities.

All versions of psychotherapy involve an interchange of ideas and emotions between the therapist and the client, with language as the medium. New narratives are thereby co-produced between therapist and client, and these provide a new template for thoughts, behaviour, and the ongoing integration of previously buried or dissociated emotions into a new, more conscious and confident self. Through exposing the patient to mild or moderate stress in a controlled environment in the process of writing these new narratives, neural growth and healing can be encouraged:

'The power of stress to trigger neural plasticity is a key element in the success of psychotherapy … As opposed to traumatic experiences, the controlled exposure to stress during therapy is a way in which therapists have attempted to harness the interaction of stress and learning in order to change the brain in a manner promoting mental health. As therapists, we work against dissociation to integrate neural networks. Integration is essentially the opposite of the dissociation observed in reaction to trauma' (pp23–24)

Central to this is the context of empathic attunement within a safe and structured environment – what Cozolino calls a '*safe emergency*' – in which clients can be encouraged to face and tolerate the anxiety of feared experience, memories and thoughts with emotional support. *'In this process',* he says, *'neural networks that are normally inhibited become activated and available for inclusion into conscious processing'* (p28).

While emphasising that therapeutic relationships can be customised to the particular needs and readiness of the individual in therapy, Cozolino is careful not to suggest that psychodynamic therapy occupies a privileged position in such encounters. Exposure in behavioural therapies and experiments in differentiation from a family systems perspective are all equally fine-tuned and focused on the making of such healing linkages in the 'safe emergency' of therapy. Indeed, he has later (Cozolino, 2006) suggested that education and ministry are equally able to use the transformative power of intimacy and language to heal the harm to the attachment system of early maladaptive experiences.

The case is thus made that, within a therapeutic setting, language and relationships are not 'mere talk', but operate on a biological plane (as we have seen, all experience does) and that the mild or moderate stress inherent in these 'safe emergencies' can stimulate neural growth and connectivity. A coherent and carefully focused new narrative can therefore heal biologically, just as medication can, and perhaps this is especially the case where co-produced between a care-giver and a patient, or 'learner'.

If this is the case, the same essential argument must then apply with equal credibility to other environments and narratives, not solely those found in the psychotherapeutic techniques, relationships and settings. While one-to-one relationships may be particularly focused, there is nothing in this argument to discount the possibility that group reinforcement and other social processes may be just as effective in helping to create and co-produce a new narrative of experience, which can then be acted upon, and so act as a similarly 'enriched environment' as focused psychotherapy.

Allan Schore has suggested that:

'The group – not only the group, but the culture – acts on and via these regulatory principals. But I would suggest that the regulatory effects of groups and cultures are much more powerful than ... the rules that cultures give. These are the ways in which human beings can pick up the emotional communications of others and can send them back out and that capacity is fundamentally affected by the early attachment relationship that is not genetically encoded. Group processes, social processes all would be acting through these and acting through the limbic system, that part of the brain which regulates emotion.' (Carroll, 2000)

This feature may then be especially significant for those services working with individuals for whom very close and personal relationships may be – perhaps from past experience – especially difficult and threatening, such as it is for people with PD. It may be, in other words, that the influence of social environments is able to go where psychotherapeutic relationships cannot. Where individuals may have chaotic and deeply charged attitudes to care-givers and figures of authority and power, it may be that the more pervasive and subtle influence of the social environment offers equally significant opportunities to engage and to encourage healing.

The potential importance of the social environment of groups, organisations and institutions of society to exacerbate or heal is therefore critical. The social environment reinforces any communication with subtle but powerful cues that go directly to our cognitive-emotional systems. Many of the most imaginative thinkers who are attempting to recognise the full significance of the plasticity of the brain are now beginning to explore the implications of social context in shaping the wiring of our brains, and therefore shaping our lives (Cohen & Stewart, 1994; Rose, 2006; Doidge, 2007; James, 2008; Gazzaniga, 2009; Gerhardt, 2010; Siegel, 2011).

Social interaction

Psychological studies and approaches, with a firm grounding in neuroscience and experimental methods, are now beginning to explore the role of social processes. These social processes operate not just at the level of whole societies and cultures and their institutions, but in more immediate, face-to-face interactions. These observations and the theorising of micro-social interactions is the territory of a branch of sociology known, appropriately, as interactionism.

In contemporary sociological theory, individuals are seen as 'social actors', constantly producing and reproducing their own version of the social world based on their expectations of themselves and others. We live, act and interact largely on the basis of our expectations of how others will act, and especially of how they will act according to how they see us. In this way, as we act upon our expectations and others act toward us in return, we are all involved in an improvised drama, which then becomes our social lives.

These social actions and expectations will, to some degree, reflect the prior life experience of the individual, and the sense of self that we bring initially to each encounter. However, the ways in which we see others – and the ways they will see us – are nevertheless limited by the generally accepted repertoire of roles, behaviours and attitudes of our social world. These social expectations as to how we should behave have a pervasive effect throughout our lives, and have a huge influence on our behaviour towards each other (Mead, 1934; Berger & Luckmann, 1966).

There seems to be a striking similarity between observations of feedback and reinforcement in social interactions with the lessons of neuroscience and the plasticity of the brain – that it is the repetition of associations we experience that strengthens the connections in our brains. In this way, the complex social worlds we inhabit are also expressed in the neural connectivity in our brains. The old distinction between nature and nurture may have been a distraction from understanding not just the unity of mind and body, but also the nature of the three-way relationship between mind, self and society (Mead, 1934; Berger & Luckmann, 1966; Dingwall *et al*, 2003). Note here that this kind of social processing effect is held to be true of all interactions, and not just those of individuals with a more conflict-prone ideation and emotion.

Sociology – like clinical psychology – is concerned with analysing the actions, behaviour and experience of the 'maladjusted' individual in terms of a series of reciprocal roles and interactions, creating and recreating the relationships. However, just as psychology's roots are in the understanding of statistically normal individuals, so this sociological account is simply one example of sociological dynamics that apply more broadly to all social interaction and our socially reaffirmed and reinforced roles and identities. For sociologists, this area is still only one aspect of 'social construction' in all areas of social life.

The particular contribution of sociology lies in the attempt to understand what is defined as problematic in any one social context. The same social action/interaction perspective that explores the production and maintenance of people's self-image through their interactions with others is then applied to studies of those interactions that take place within the organisations and institutions in society that manage the behaviour of individuals who present some kind of 'social problem', such as those with PD or complex trauma. For these more organised and structured interactions, we need another level of analysis.

The role of institutions in social reinforcement

There is, for current purpose, little distinction between civil society and social practice; we use it here to mean the organised matrix of activities for social purposes that encounter and work with individuals under stress, with past or present trauma, and/or with formal psychiatric illness. They may do so as a specialist focus, or simply among all the other people that they encounter in their ordinary day-to-day activity. It is the broader purpose, and the degree of organisation, that defines the territory.

It is the sociologists – very loosely defined – who have gone furthest in trying to unravel the life course of interactions between individuals (especially more vulnerable, challenging or chaotic individuals) and the 'others' whom they meet, not just in spontaneous interactions but in formal roles and with codified responsibilities, in organisations, where the rules of engagement and the 'definition of the situation' is determined by the organisation as such (Becker, 1963; Goffman, 1959; 1971; Berger & Luckmann, 1966; Schur, 1971; Matza, 1964; 1969).

Here, the particular contribution of sociology has been to take as much interest in the actions, expectations and self-fulfilling prophecies of the staff as they do in the 'service users' themselves (Baruch & Treacher, 1978; Prior, 1993). The dysfunctional self-image and behaviour of the individual is only one part of the analysis; the reaction of 'others' is equally a subject for study (Lemert, 1951; Berne, 1964; Laing & Esterson, 1964; Henry, 1972; Scheff, 1999; Cromby, 2004; 2005). For example, in the sociology of the management of 'deviance', the attitudes and beliefs of staff are seen as having a significant impact upon the course and outcome of dysfunctional behaviour (Lemert 1951; Prior, 1993; Clinard & Meier, 2011).

There has been relatively little sociological study of social interactions in relation to PD and complex needs (but see Daniels, 1970; Manning, 2001). Nevertheless, the various studies from social science seem to challenge the immediate assumption that any fixity of behaviour is the result of characteristics of the individual. Society's institutions are at least equally powerful themselves in moulding the behaviour and the self-image of the individuals they manage. These approaches suggest the need to consider more critically the role of treatment or other remedial agencies (Illich *et al*, 1977; Ingleby, 1981).

Many earlier studies in the sociological tradition also explored the extent to which tensions within the organisation of services may partly account for the inability of agencies to respond more constructively (Stanton & Schwartz, 1954; Goffman, 1961; Sudnow, 1967; Barton, 1976; Box, 1971; Woodhouse & Pengelly, 1991; Cabinet Office, 2006). Such sociological or ethnographic analyses are then complemented by studies of the functioning of organisations from a psychodynamic perspective, to which we now turn.

Chapter 4
Socio-emotional systems

Robin Johnson

Individual change and systematic change

To recap, the jury may be out over how far the maladaptive behaviour characteristic of personality disorder (PD) and complex trauma is essentially embedded in the personality through early trauma in critical development periods, or how far it remains malleable through constructive, containing and enabling experiences, in social interactions later in life.

Both the 'hard' and 'soft' evidence (that is, the neurobiological and the psycho-social) indicate that attachment difficulties, emotional disregulation and poor social problem-solving underlie many emotional and behavioural issues. In more severe cases they also underlie many diagnoses of PD or complex trauma.

The frustrating, self-defeating, dysfunctional and emotional world of the individual with PD – and to a lesser extent, of us all – may at least in part reflect the way that the infant brain has developed at an early stage, in a hostile and unresponsive, traumatising emotional environment. However, it may also be in part due to such individuals' greater reliance later in life on a limited and inflexible repertoire of responses to stress, exacerbated by the beliefs and feelings underlying such behavioural repertoires.

In other words, we have a vicious circle, or feedback loop, in which an individual's response in a given situation might be limited by their previous experiences, ensuring his or her behaviour follows the same pattern. In that respect, such behaviour reflects, just as much as it creates, the powerful dynamism of re-enactment of such early traumatic schemas, which tends to evoke punitive or rejecting responses in others, so perpetuating rather than breaking the reinforcement cycle. However, the very process of re-enacting behaviour serves to strengthen the related emotional and neurological connections, thus completing the circle and ensuring that the next time a similar situation arises, they are likely to respond in the same manner.

These are not, however, questions, options and hypotheses that are easily tested in laboratory conditions. Granted the multiplicity of perspectives and the uncertain corroboration between findings based on quite different methods and paradigms (Rose, 2005), it has been suggested that only empirical evidence from 'naturalistic studies' (Dolan & Coid, 1995) may be able to confirm the balance of factors. With relatively few individuals engaging effectively with treatment services, this approach may be just as meaningful as studies of the relative efficacy of different treatment approaches (Fonagy, 2004).

One key question is how far the failure to evoke more constructive experiences may actually be exacerbated as a consequence of unintentional mismanagement of these social and emotional conflicts by others involved – by care-givers, welfare and correction agencies. To ask this is not to lay blame – as we shall see, these self-perpetuating patterns can be very hard to intercept – but simply to ask aloud the question that many will already be asking themselves: did we get it right? Did we help?

Here, therefore, we begin to move from an understanding of biology and neuroscience, and of social science and psychotherapy, to studies of the actual practice of organisations. One question that we must now address, is what may interrupt the development of positive encounters from well-crafted services to meet such widespread and pressing needs?

Effecting change within the individual

What evidence there is certainly suggests that personal change work is genuinely a harder task with and for those with histories of PD and complex trauma. Clinicians' and other frontline services' reports alike tell of the difficulty of 'getting it right', and much of the evidence for a capacity to change remains problematic. The evidence from healthcare on standard clinical/therapeutic interventions for specific PDs is especially equivocal.

However, it is still incompatible with the sweeping 'therapeutic nihilism' of the past. There is now good evidence that even severely traumatised individuals – those with, for example, a formal diagnosis of PD – do have the capacity to respond to therapeutic and other interventions, as long as they are crafted with care to respond to the underlying problems and not just the surface presentation.

Where more standard approaches such as medication, counselling or behavioural therapy alone have proven less effective, it may be necessary to enlist a wider and more creative range of influences and interventions in support of the therapeutic or remedial task. More treatment-derived evidence on attachment and recovery, whether from a psychiatric or a psychological or systems psychodynamic framework, tends to stress that the therapeutic encounter or setting must be able to engage and contain the emotional charge presented by the individual's distress (Winnicott, 1965; Bowlby, 1988; Menzies, 1990; Department of Health/NIMHE, 2003b; Gerhardt, 2004; Johnson, 1981; Dartington, 2010; Barrett, 2011).

Tasks and emotions in social systems

Social systems as defences against anxiety

Our next port of call in observing social practice may therefore be to revisit the social systems (or 'socio-emotional systems') analysis developed recently, as a development within the psychodynamic tradition.

Elliott Jaques, a Canadian psychoanalyst and organisational psychologist, first proposed the concept of social systems as defences against unconscious anxiety (Jaques, 1953). Jaques took up the idea that there could be unconscious dynamic processes within a group (eg. Bion, 1961) – now being called, therefore, group dynamics – just as there are within an individual's own mind, and he applied these ideas more broadly to organisations as a whole.

Jaques argued that there was likely to be a close relationship between the objective and practical aims of an organisation (ie. the treatment of patients) and these emotions and largely unconscious group dynamics, and that each can support or distort and undermine the other. Where they support each other, you have an exceptionally successful organisation in which the members will always go the extra mile. Where they conflict, there will be friction and inefficiencies, with tensions acted out in sickness rates, industrial relations conflicts, delays, complaints etc.

Jaques' interest then was not confined to psychotherapy, but rather he sought to explore difficulties in, for example, an industrial work force. His work was primarily a contribution to another growing field – occupational psychology. However, his ideas, combined with those of many others in the Tavistock Institute group (De Board, 1978; Trist & Murray, 1990; Shapiro & Carr, 1991; Obholzer & Zagier Roberts, 1994; Hirschhorn, 1997; Hinshelwood & Skogstad, 2000; Huffington & Armstrong, 2004; Dartington, 2010) have remained as an undercurrent in social science and organisational consultancy.

The suggestion is now coming from many different quarters that we need to more closely examine the ways in which actual groups, organisations and institutions – civil society in this broader sense – operate to manage effectively or badly the emotional life of their members. This should be important for the healthy functioning and efficiency of any organisation, from a purely commercial operation to one with education, welfare or correction at its heart. However, it may be especially important for organisations that must – willingly or otherwise – spend much of their time with individuals who show the signs of stress, trauma and disorder.

Socio-emotional systems analysis in a care setting

Isobel Menzies, a nurse and colleague of Jaques, trained in psychoanalytic and group dynamic interpretations, had originally been called in to advise on a problem in nursing training at a teaching hospital. Every year about one-third of student nurses failed to complete the course and left. There was some concern that ward duties might be being given precedence over the students' training needs and Menzies was asked to investigate.

Menzies (1990) found that the drop-out rate among students was really only one expression of tensions within the organisation of the hospital and in the ward staffing. The disaffection and demoralisation of the students on placement reflected wider problems, and should be read as a warning sign, rather like canaries in a mine used to detect gas. The drop-out rate for students expressed, in an oblique way, the emotional difficulties that were undermining the work of the unit as a whole.

Menzies observed that the unit was exposing the nursing staff, on a daily basis, to huge emotional challenges and conflicts. They were expected to work with often highly intimate bodily functions, blood and faeces, and yet maintain an unemotional, practical demeanour. Patients, sometimes severely ill, might die; others who recovered would simply disappear. In either case, there might be relatives to deal with, and anxieties and issues of their own.

The operational policies for the nursing staff appeared designed to minimise this emotional charge by creating emotional distance between the nurses and the patients. Nurses were given a few specialised tasks, which they carried out with large numbers of patients. This kind of industrial specialisation might appear to be efficient, but in practice it restricted human contact between nurse and patient. The nurses therefore adopted a way of managing their work tasks and only indirectly talking about the patient, thus depersonalising the work – they would talk of 'the liver in bed 16', for example, or 'the dressings in bed seven'.

At the same time, in order to efficiently manage the responsibilities and risks of even menial tasks with such vulnerable individuals, every activity was reported, checked and double-checked. Tasks were 'delegated up' through the nursing and ward hierarchy, so that nurses were often doing work that gave no recognition of their degree of experience and might be well below their competence. As a result, an atmosphere grew in which nurses were reluctant to take initiatives or make decisions over their own time or in recognition of patient's needs, while guidelines restricted any exercise of delegation or discretion. They were trying to work as part angel, part automata.

However, in practice this meant that the nursing staff were constantly exposed to emotional challenges in their relationships with their patients, from anxiety to embarrassment, grief and frustration, and yet they had no scope or opportunity to deal with these. These ineffective and counterproductive ways to keep the emotional content of their work at bay seemed simply to lead to high stress and low morale. Bureaucratic and professional defences against the emotional content of the work were just not working.

Being a psychoanalyst by training, Menzies' approach did not involve simply walking in, observing, identifying the problem, writing a report for the management with recommendations, and leaving. Instead, she spent many months working with the nursing staff and hospital management, to win their trust, help them discover between them the issues that were disturbing them, and help them work through how they might operate differently and come up with their own solutions (Lawlor & Webb, 2009). As a result, the hospital introduced new nursing and patient management practices that worked to reconcile the emotional and the practical aspects of their work, and the papers that Menzies wrote began to redefine the nature and role of nursing as a profession.

In her later work on a childcare ward, Menzies was one of a number of influential researchers, alongside Bowlby, Ainsworth and the Roberstons, who transformed the way we now manage infant care in hospital, putting care for the emotional needs of the child on a par with physical care.

The kind of social system analysis that Jaques, Menzies and others in the Tavistock school pioneered was quickly taken up in psychiatric care.

In Section three we will return to explore the history of these developments, and current attempts to revive the recognition of emotional intelligence in services.

The influence of Menzies' study

A number of very important long-term conclusions were drawn from the Menzies study and a generation of further investigations of the emotional lives of organisations.

First, the solutions to hidden emotional conflicts within the organisation came from recognising the human reality of relationships and emotions, and then setting out to change the way the organisation worked, to manage not just those emotions but the basic task – in Menzies' case, nursing and acute care – more humanely, and hence more effectively. Attempts to remove the personal element from personal services assume that procedures can be 'manualised' and mechanised without the loss of the most important elements. This can create a false economy that is at odds with the true nature of the work.

To some extent this issue has been recognised recently, at least in the understanding of the importance of leadership in schools and in prisons (Liebling & Arnold, 2004). It might even be argued that recent calls for the recognition of the importance of social capital, and even for the creation of what some are calling a 'Big Society', reflect the need to acknowledge the importance of relationships and relational health (Jordan, 2001; Frey *et al*, 2005; Johnson & Haigh, 2011b). There have at least been suggestions that no public health agenda that ignores the emotional and mental health of the population can hope to make any headway (Royal College of Psychiatrists, 2010).

The second important conclusion drawn from the study was that those changes that Menzies' work fostered came from working with the staff team rather than imposing a managerial solution, such as a restructuring, from the outside. When we find a situation that is not working, we cannot assume that the answer lies simply in importing new and supposedly more efficient processes from elsewhere. These tend to produce at best a veneer of change, and at worst are simply a distraction, even a form of displacement activity, that obscures the issues. The possible exception here is the importing of more inspirational leadership – but even here, leadership is only effective when working with the organisation and the people in it as whole, rather than simply bringing in a new model and then rapidly moving on.

Change that really involves all participants in exploring new ways to work will not only be better informed, but also better motivated. In the case of acute hospital care, the emotions of the patients themselves are a significant element, though it may not be appropriate to expect them to be involved in a redesign of the service. In other contexts, however, the wishes and views of the patients (or service users) may also be a very relevant and useful input.

Further implications of Menzies' study

There are, however, two further implications of Menzies' study, which are particularly relevant to future generations – that is to say, our own – rather than to the organisational and professional cultures of the immediate post-war era.

First, we have seen the introduction over the past 20 years or more of a management philosophy in care services, education etc that does not look to the providers of services to innovate, but accentuates instead either the client (as 'customer') or the local commissioners of services. However, there is clearly still a risk that services will be 'purchased' or 'commissioned', and their 'outcomes' measured, according to quite superficial and simplistic measures – a return to the organisation's supposed aims with no thought to the emotional and group dynamics that make for real quality.

The extent to which the 'purchaser/provider split' has in itself created an awkward and potentially dysfunctional relationship between services and commissioners is currently a major concern (Ballat and Campling, 2011). A tendency to excessive interference or 'micro-management' of frontline services has not only restricted the scope for creativity and responsiveness of services, and contributed to lower morale and job satisfaction, it has also, by its over specification of services, demanded more senior-management time in tendering and monitoring, and so actually produced less efficiency (House of Commons, 2010).

The second novel element concerns the tendency in recent years to regard emotion and psychology as issues of mental health, and therefore the preserve of the expert, whether to be vested in human resources divisions of the organisation or in specialist 'therapeutic interventions' from skilled mental health professionals. Menzies' work – and that of Jaques before her, and the many others who have come after – demonstrated the need to return emotional intelligence to the workforce. Once we assume that the recognition of human sensitivity requires a referral to a specialist service, we simply further disempower our frontline staff.

This is not to say that there is no role for specialist skills, but that the proper role of specialists here is to support ordinary people in ordinary situations to find their own best solutions. This is a theme that we will find again and again in the practice examples that are the focus of the next section of this book.

Distorted self-images in individuals and interactions

At this point, we need to consider one key aspect of the experience of individuals with distorted self-images: the phenomenon known as 'ego-syntonicity'.

Both social psychology and sociology tend to suggest that an individual's characteristics may be more responsive to social processes than they may initially seem, but that social interactions tend to reinforce set expectations and the social roles and repertoires of the individual. Moreover, as the range of responses of individuals diagnosable with PD is typically more restricted, more extreme, less sensitive or nuanced, certainly more demanding or disruptive, it is then perhaps understandable and entirely natural for blame and social rejection to result in identifying the individual rather than the interaction as the principal determining feature, and therefore the source.

This tendency to locate the issues in the individual applies also to the experience of the individual at the centre of these interactions themselves. The behaviours that are characteristic of individuals with PD arise from the individuals' sense of themselves – their 'ego'. Their behaviour therefore appears entirely natural and normal to the individual concerned; it is not experienced as external, alien or distinct from ordinary experience – which indeed, for the individual, they are not. In other words, the individual suffering from PD cannot imagine a different way of being or thinking, or that things will ever change.

The term 'ego-syntonicity' was coined to describe distorted perceptions of the self that nevertheless seem entirely consistent, plausible and acceptable (or 'syntonic') to the individual. It is a phenomenon seen in other psychiatric conditions such as anorexia, or body dysmorphia. However, this aspect of ego-syntonicity is also characteristic of PD, and it is one of the key features that distinguishes PD and complex trauma from many other psychiatric phenomena such as panic states, flashbacks, mood swings or hallucinations.

This self reinforcing, ongoing cognitive/affective consonance can actually be linked to recent neuroscience findings (LeDoux, 1998; Panksepp, 1998) that indicate that emotions and perceptions are much more closely intertwined than rationalist philosophers have tended to allow for (Shotter, 1993; Pert, 1998; Damasio, 1999; Carroll, 2000; Cromby, 2005). However, it can also be linked to repetitive re-enactment in social settings, where the self-perpetuating reinforcement is either strengthened or weakened, hence suggesting that different management can make a difference.

This then highlights the potential of adopting new roles in a social context – which is the basis of a lot of socio-therapeutic work – and leads on naturally to the potential benefits to be found in environments (such as hostels and other homelessness community networks, and substance abuse support services) where some form of peer support or mentoring is developed.

This syntonicity tends to deter people from seeking help, or at least from seeking help for the underlying problem. It may also be the reason why services working with and supporting individuals with the more deeply entrenched forms of complex trauma – whether as children or as adults – need to pay particular attention to consistency, coherence and clarity in their work. It may be one of the reasons why approaches such as the therapeutic community (Main, 1946), nidotherapy (Tyrer & Kramo, 2007), re-parenting, and other 'wrap-around' environments (Batmanghelidjh, 2006) may be effective – a reflection of the need to have all the 'messages' and cues in the immediate social environment reinforcing the intended outcomes of the treatment (Carroll, 2000).

It may also help us to grasp why, for those on the fringes of treatment or other services who are deeply wary or ambivalent at best over accepting help, services tend to create stepwise or staged engagement to gradually build up trust, engagement and relationships.

Section two

Innovations in practice

Section two:

Innovations in practice

Introduction

The central section of this book illustrates the themes, theories and arguments outlined in Section one with examples drawn from the world of practice. Here, many hundreds and thousands of workers and carers are developing new approaches in their everyday lives that recognise, consciously or unconsciously, the significance of traumatising experience, and the need to respond creatively and constructively to the challenges of disruptive emotions.

The section covers a wide territory that includes:

- playwork with children in a Romanian orphanage
- a debating society for youngsters excluded from school
- counselling for residents in a hostel for rough sleepers and ex-offenders
- a telephone hotline for servicemen at risk of combat stress, and a self-build housing project for ex-servicemen
- peer support for occupational stress in the fire service
- a community enterprise for people with drug and alcohol histories.

They all demonstrate creative and innovative ways of working with the after-effects of trauma – some explicit, others not, some involving early intervention, others only very much later down the line. Between them they offer a narrative on trauma throughout life. All have more in common than we might at first glance expect, and far more than our fragmented imaginations often allow us to see.

In some cases, the primary focus is on a personal relationship – with a keyworker for example, or a psychotherapist, a helpline counsellor or peer mentor. In most cases, this personal relationship is effective because it is embedded in a carefully planned and supportive environment. The wider social networks – and especially the network of peers – also have a major role to play in many of these examples, and perhaps in the long run the most important role in the whole experience.

We start by looking at work with children and young people, and focus on the kind of early intervention services that are often now commended, and are considered to be effective in tackling the effects of abuse and neglect. It has recently been argued (Allen & Duncan Smith, 2010; Marmot, 2009) that such early intervention is critical to tackle the wider and long-term impact of trauma on health and social exclusion.

As the section progresses we focus on later interventions, once the aftermath of any earlier failure has begun to have a significant and pervasive impact on individuals' lives. These chapters look at ways in which intervention during these still formative stages should also be seen as preventive. Still other examples consider the services and approaches that are being developed to intervene and support when trauma threatens late in life. The similarity in some of the themes here with those for early trauma is, we propose, further food for thought.

The neuroscience of trauma now shows us, with greater scientific precision, what in truth we always knew: that the emotional environment in which a child is raised can cause enormous harm. Yet there are equally important insights to be drawn from contemporary practice, and especially in pioneering initiatives both in therapy and in other forms of remedial work that would not regard themselves as therapy. The need for theory and practice to inform each other is one of the themes for the future that we explore in the concluding section.

All these practice examples, and the rationale for their inclusion, have something to tell us about the ongoing interaction between trauma and the social environment, and the extent to which socio-therapeutic or 'enabling' environments can be mobilised to support the task of recovery.

Editor's comment:

Playwork and recovery potential

It is common to see young children, as they explore and act out the dramas of their lives, as 'just playing', as if play is a trivial and inconsequential thing. However, play is the essential means by which we, as a species, explore the social world.

Infancy is a time of fundamental formative learning – but also for un-learning. The role and potential of playwork to liberate a traumatised child, or equally to enable a damaged adult to explore new relationships, via music, for example, cannot be seen solely in terms of the acquisition of certain skills.

In 2005, playwork researchers Fraser Brown and Sophie Webb published an article – Children without play – which described a small-scale research study conducted during the first year of a playwork intervention with abandoned children living in a Romanian paediatric hospital. These children, kept in conditions of shocking neglect, had been assumed to be 'retarded' and were simply warehoused while awaiting transfer to an adult institution.

Their article highlights the dramatic improvements seen in these children over the remarkably short period of the playwork project. It quotes extensively from reflective diaries kept by one of the authors in the course of their work in order to identify some of the most significant therapeutic elements of playwork.

The article interweaves this account with observations on the striking parallels between the behaviour patterns of these children and those exhibited by infant monkeys reared in isolation in research conducted in the 1950s and 60s by Harry Harlow and his team. This research has been widely publicised and has been highly influential in our understanding of the role of attachment in human development. Far less well known are some of the other studies Harlow and his team undertook, which are explored in the article, now reproduced in edited form in the following chapter.

If it is the case that, when critical periods of development in the infant brain are missed or disturbed, such as by traumatising experiences of abuse and neglect, then the brain will be chronically impaired and behavioural problems will develop later in life as a consequence, then we should expect the neglected children in this study to have a very limited capacity to respond.

The findings of the study suggest otherwise. This research convincingly demonstrates the importance of play, not merely as an aid to normal development, but as a means to recovery and healthy development for seriously and chronically neglected and deprived children.

This was a very small scale study, in less than ideal conditions for formal research. There is no random sample, no control group, no double blind. There are, however, mercifully few naturally occurring experimental situations like this from which to learn about child development and responsiveness.

However, these findings suggest that:

1. We can never write off children, or adults, as too damaged to recover.
2. It is all too easy to attribute the consequences of institutionalised neglect and blindness to the characteristics of the victims.
3. We must never cease to learn from actual practice.

Chapter 5
Children without play

Fraser Brown and Sophie Webb[1]

Some years ago, the authors undertook a small scale research study examining the impact of a playwork project on a group of abandoned children living in a Romanian paediatric hospital (Webb & Brown, 2003). The children, ranging in age from one to ten years old, had suffered chronic neglect and abuse. They had previously spent most of their lives tied in the same cot in the same hospital ward day after day, some for many years, and for most of their lives. They were poorly fed and their nappies were rarely changed. Although able to see and hear other children, they experienced little in the way of social interaction.

The playwork project started in the summer of 1999 and continues today. It started as a result of the concern of the newly appointed Director of the Sighisoara Paediatric Hospital, Dr Cornel Puscas. When confronted with a ward full of disturbed children sitting rocking in their own solitary worlds, he was reminded of one of the most powerful conclusions from Harlow's studies: *'Play is of utmost importance for the subsequent social well-being of the individual and those around him'* (Suomi & Harlow, 1971).

Hoping to help the children recover some sort of 'normality', he approached the White Rose Initiative (WRI), a Leeds-based charity, for funding to employ someone to play with the children. They employed Edit Bus, the first ever Romanian playworker, and brought her to Leeds Metropolitan University for a specially designed training course. Upon her return to Romania, Edit worked with the children for four months before being joined by Sophie Webb for an extended period, and later by Fraser Brown for briefer periods.

During a period when nothing changed in their lives other than their introduction to the playwork project, the children themselves changed

---

1 The following article first appeared in the *Journal of Education* (2005) **35** pp139–158.

dramatically: their social interaction became more complex; physical activity showed a distinct move from gross to fine motor skills; the children's understanding of the world around them was improved; and they began to play in highly creative ways. They no longer sat rocking and staring vacantly into space, but instead they had become fully engaged and active human beings.

During the first year of the WRI project, the two Leeds Met researchers spent more than 500 hours working with Edit, and studying this small group of children. Our original intention was to help alleviate the suffering of the children, but it quickly became apparent that remarkable changes were occurring. We therefore resolved to conduct a research study of the outcomes of the playwork project, to observe the children's play development and assess developmental change during the first year of the project. It was possible to observe the children each day, noting the details of their play behaviours and social interactions. In this article, we will attempt to identify some of the most significant therapeutic elements of playwork from our detailed analysis of the play behaviours of this unique group of children.

Methods of participant observation

In the early stages of the study we adopted a form of participant observation where the participant's role is partially concealed. Our observations had to be unobtrusive for two reasons: first, to avoid disrupting what the children were achieving in their play, and second, to enable the recording of detailed notes at close quarters. Although our dual role was understood by the Romanian playworker and the director of the hospital, everyone else would have seen us as visiting playworkers from the UK. In the later stages of the study we employed a slightly different observation technique ie. rotated peer observation, which saw us alternating tasks and roles – one hour working with the children, one hour of non-participant observation, and vice versa.

However, it is our view that the role of the playworker is particularly suited to participant observation. It is one of the guiding principles of playwork that the child's agenda should be regarded as the starting point for child-adult interactions (Hughes, 1996). This means that playworkers naturally adopt an approach that encourages them as researchers to avoid dominating the adult-child relationship. This is also reflected in a second guiding principle of playwork, namely, 'negative capability' (Fisher, 2002), which will be discussed later.

An effective playworker expects to pick up on signals rather than instigate them, which means that they are adopting an approach similar to that of the classic Tavistock Model (Greig & Taylor, 1999). This encourages researchers to interact with the subjects and record the behaviours and feelings of all the participants, including themselves. In the Romanian context, we made extensive use of reflective diaries, not simply as a memory aid but also to provide raw data. The following diary extract, which was written after Sophie's first visit to the hospital, illustrates the approach.

'***The silence.*** *Every room was full of children in cots, but it was so quiet. Even when we entered the room there was no sound from the children. They just looked at us. The smell of urine in every room was almost unbearable.* ***The emptiness.*** *Each room had just the cots with plastic mattresses. The children were dirty and wearing clothes that were too big for them. Some were wearing jumpers as trousers, and none of them were wearing shoes. There were rags around their waists, which I later found out were ripped up sheets tied to keep the nappies in place. These rags were also used to tie the children to the cots. Most children were sitting rocking and others were standing up banging the sides of their cots against the walls. Giving the children a cuddle was strange as they either held on too tightly, or they remained stiff and unfeeling.'* (Reflective Diary, 6 February 2000)

Our assessments of the children's progress were made using a variation on a system developed during an earlier study of children's play behaviours (Brown, 2003). The children were assessed at three stages, in February, April and August 2000, using the questions in the assessment tool that we had developed. There was evidence of change in all the children, albeit to differing degrees, which may reflect a combination of their individual make-up and their life experience. This was extremely encouraging in terms of its implications for the recovery potential of abused and neglected children. It was also slightly chilling, since the medical records described most of the children as 'retarded'.

We were told informally, although this was not confirmed in the medical records, that most of them were waiting for places in a children's mental hospital. Thankfully, their remarkable progress meant that 14 of the original 16 children were eventually either adopted or fostered. Sadly the other two were eventually transferred to a children's mental hospital. It has not been possible to conduct any longitudinal follow-up on the children.

For the purposes of this article it is sufficient to restate our conclusion: that the children's developmental progress was clearly identifiable, and apparently made possible through their experience of the playwork project.

The nature of playwork

Some readers may be new to the concept of playwork, so we are including here a few words of explanation. Playwork is rooted in an understanding that children learn and develop through their play. There are, nevertheless, many instances in modern society where that process is interrupted or impaired. Playwork involves not just playing, but also identifying and removing barriers to the play process, and enriching the child's play environment.

Playwork is thus a generic term for a profession that encompasses those occupations where the medium of play is used as the major mechanism for redressing aspects of developmental imbalance (Brown and Webb, 2002). This may be something as straightforward as providing an after-school club for children who would otherwise have nowhere to play, or something as complex as creating an environment to assist the recovery of children who have suffered severe deprivation.

Prior to the start of the playwork project, the Romanian group appear to have experienced an unpredictable combination of both these forms of play deprivation. They were deprived as a result of being tied in their cots for most of the day, with virtually no social interaction, but they were also treated in an erratic way by the nurses, who might feed them properly one day but forget to feed them the next.

It is one of the most basic assumptions of the playwork profession that, given the right conditions, children will learn and develop through their play. It is the role of a playworker to create those conditions, so that the play process can be effective. Depending on local circumstances this could mean anything from feeding hungry children and changing their nappies, to providing toys and craft materials in order for them to explore their own creativity. The project workers in Romania did all those things.

Ultimately, the aim of playwork is to provide an environment that enables the child to grow towards self-fulfilment, referred to by Maslow (1971) as self-actualisation.

Enriched play environments and child development

The playworker's initial role is to analyse the child's environment in order to identify and remove any barriers to the play process. In most playwork projects there are elements of the work that have little to do with play, but which nevertheless have to be addressed, otherwise the quality of the child's play experience is likely to be restricted. For example, checking the safety of play equipment on an adventure playground is not in itself a playful activity, but most playworkers regard it as part of their role.

Given the extreme levels of neglect and deprivation in the orphanage, the issue of 'barriers to play' was far more significant than might be encountered in most UK settings. While the Romanian project involved a range of elements, from basic human care to highly complex therapeutic play, we regard most of the tasks performed by the workers as crucial to the playwork role.

The playworker is concerned with enriching the child's play environment in order to stimulate the play process. However, enriching the play environment is not so much about aiding specific elements of learning, but adopting a holistic approach to learning. There are a number of factors that playworkers have to take into account when considering how best to create such an environment. For the purposes of our research study we grouped them under 11 subheadings:

- freedom
- flexibility
- socialisation and social interaction
- physical activity
- intellectual stimulation
- creativity and problem solving
- emotional equilibrium
- self-discovery

- ethical stance
- adult/child relationships
- general appeal (eg. humour, colour etc).

The following extracts illustrate the way in which the playworker's gentle interaction helped to stimulate the children and enable them to take control of their own environment:

'I found some feathers in the cupboard today and went around tickling them ... Virgil was really afraid at first and threw his arms up shouting, but when I tickled my own arm and showed him it was okay – he was more curious. The look on his face when he felt comfortable to feel the feather was absolutely beautiful ... so fresh and innocent.' (Reflective Diary, 17 February 2000)

'Today I sat Elena on the car and she stayed there, so I showed Carol how to push her and then they were able to do it on their own! I think it was a real step for Elena, as she never 'plays' with the others she just touches them every so often. Until today this was her play ... a beginning that needed nurturing?' (Reflective Diary, 24 March 2000)

It is in such observations of the subtle minutiae of an individual child's responses, as captured in the diaries, that the opportunities for growth may come.

For many playworkers the most important element in their work is compound flexibility ie. *'the interrelationship between a flexible/adaptable environment and the gradual development of flexibility/adaptability in the child'* (Brown, 2003), to encourage 'adaptive variability' (Sutton-Smith, 1997). Taking these two concepts together we can infer that the role of the playworker is to create flexible environments that are substantially adaptable or controllable by the children.

The following extract illustrates the way in which children made use of the inherent flexibility of a box (actually a rubbish bin) to create two games of their own.

'While Ion was sitting in a big yellow box, Virgil started to play a game with him involving an imaginary object. He pretended to receive something from Edit and then took it back to Ion in the box, who took it from him

and put it in his lap. The spontaneous interaction between them both was fascinating to watch. Afterwards Virgil continued playing with the yellow plastic box, by putting it on his head and walking around the room ... He created a sort of obstacle course out of the cots and tables.'
(Reflective Diary, 25 February 2000)

Negative capability

Most adults who come into contact with children bring their own agenda to that relationship. For example, teachers have an obligation to teach the national curriculum. Doctors, social workers, even parents, invariably have their own adult priorities. The playworker is unusual in that he or she attempts to suspend personal prejudice, and go along with the flow of the children's needs and tastes.

This brings us to the concept of 'negative capability' mentioned previously. The poet John Keats suggested that this was a characteristic of all creative minds. He recommended the complete suspension of all prejudices and preconceptions as a prelude to opening up the creative flow of the mind. The similarity between this approach to creativity and one of the most fundamental aspects of the child-adult relationship in playwork was identified by Fisher (2002). She suggested that playworkers have to guard against entering the play environment with their own preconceptions and prejudices; only then will they truly be there for the child. This approach requires a great sensitivity to the learning potential of the playwork setting, and means the playworker has to be prepared to stand back when others might be inclined to rush in:

'The children do fight a lot and I only intervene if it gets too violent or if I can see they won't work it out themselves. I think they learn more from their own reactions than from adults at times and it's good for them to work out their own disagreements.' (Reflective Diary, 22 March 2000)

For the playworker in a therapeutic setting it is especially important to take the child's agenda as the starting point for interactions. In the child's daily life, play is their only experience of being in control of events. If playworkers are not to 'adulterate' that experience, they have to ensure that, wherever possible, they are following the child's agenda (Else and Sturrock, 1998). It follows that in most circumstances the playworker would expect to adopt an approach of *'preparation followed by withdrawal'* (Hughes, 1996).

The Romanian children required a stronger presence over a more extended period, but it remained the case that most of our interventions were a response to the specific play behaviours of each child. The following example refers to a ten-year-old child who was too frightened to walk independently. He was obsessed with shoes, and the playworker was able to work with that with dramatic results:

'I have played 'shoes' with Nicolae for the past two weeks and that appears to have led him to trust me. Today, after playing 'shoes' yet again, I stood him in the middle of the room, about four steps away from me. Usually he just sits down, but this time he walked towards me with his arms stretched out for a hug. I think these may have been his first independent steps (after 10 years!).' (Reflective Diary, 24 February 2000)

One of the most significant elements of the playwork role is the way in which relationships are made with the children. If the child-adult relationship is effective, there is a good chance of not only helping children with their problems, but also of raising their self-esteem generally. For example, a child who spends most of the time throwing stones around may simply be a 'trajectory' child who has been offered no other way of connecting with his/her basic schema. A playworker who provides a set of skittles, or a game of cricket, may be able to address the situation effectively, without recourse to disciplinary controls. In the playground setting, an 'enclosing' child might be stimulated by opportunities to build dens; a 'rotater' might like the roundabout etc. By responding to these favoured schemata we are giving the child a powerful message, that we respect what matters to them. By so doing, the playworker can help to build the child's self-esteem. For example:

'Virgil was happy about playing with the crayons, he was laughing about taking them out of the box and putting them in again. He likes doing this more than using them to colour in! He does it with other toys he plays with, always has to tidy!' (Reflective Diary, 22 February 2000)

Cultural understanding

Besides knowledge based on child development, therapeutic playworkers need to have 'cultural competence' – of their own and others' cultures. Here we are not simply referring to the need to understand and respect the culture of a different race or religion, but there are also 'cultures within cultures'.

Thus, in the Romanian example, it was not only important to develop an understanding of national characteristics, but also the culture of the local town and the paediatric hospital itself. Even the nurses on the abandoned children's ward had their own culture, which had to be respected otherwise life could be made very difficult. Here is an extreme example of the lengths that we had to go to in order to be allowed to stay and work with these children:

'I think the hardest part of the day for me is having to put them back in their cots again, but it will create even more aggravation if I don't, and that could ruin everything. People would probably think I'm awful for doing it, but I've had to accept that this is part of their system whether I like it or not. I know the nurses will tie them back in after we leave.' (Reflective Diary, 25 February 2000)

On a positive note, the longer term impact of the WRI project has been considerable: the nurses stopped tying the children to their cots during the second year of the project; the children are now well fed; their nappies are changed regularly and the hospital has recently adopted a policy of finding abandoned children foster placements within six months.

Ethological parallels

The antecedents of the playwork project are interesting to explore, as they highlight some striking parallels with a well-known series of ethological studies conducted by Harry Harlow during the 1950s and 1960s. Harlow's experiments were summarised in the article 'Monkeys without play' (Suomi and Harlow, 1971), the conclusion being that *'monkey play is of overwhelming importance'*, and that the same must be true of human play. For this reason, Harlow's experiments have generally been considered to have great significance for playworkers.

In Harlow's laboratory, infant monkeys were raised in a variety of ways. Some were left with the mother and allowed to play with peers, and this group showed no developmental differences from monkeys raised in the wild. Others were raised by the mother, but given no peer interaction, resulting in these infants developing disturbing patterns of behaviour as they matured. Another group of infants was isolated from their mothers but allowed to play with their peers. As long as they also experienced some form of 'contact comfort', this group developed normally. The tactile input might be something as simple as a piece of soft cloth, and the play input might be as little as half an hour a day. This led Leonard Rosenblum, one of Harlow's collaborators, to suggest that *'there are three variables to love – touch, motion, and play – and if you can supply all of those, you are meeting a primate's needs'* (Slater, 2004).

However, Harlow's experiments did not stop there. A further group of infant monkeys were raised in cages where they were able to see and hear other monkeys but not able to play with them, or interact in any meaningful way. Not surprisingly in such circumstances, the monkeys developed clear signs of disturbed behaviour. Harlow found that when his infant monkeys were introduced to peers, they did not seem able to play. Rather, *'they avoid social interchange and continue in their self-directed, self-satisfying behaviours'* (Suomi and Harlow, 1971). Thus:

'Having no mother or peers to cling to, these monkeys embrace their own bodies in intensive self-clasping. Having no maternal nipple to suckle, they suck and chew their own digits ... Having no playmates to provide motor stimulation, wire-cage reared infants develop compulsive and stereotypic rocking behaviours, strikingly reminiscent of the human autistic child.' (Suomi and Harlow, 1971)

It is this group that we are particularly interested in. The parallels between the two sets of primates (monkey and human) are obvious. The Romanian children had also lived most of their lives trapped behind bars (in this case, their cots), in a hospital ward where they could see and hear other infants, but could not play with them. At the beginning of the playwork project the children exhibited many similar behaviour patterns to those identified by Harlow. When untied, fed and bathed, and then taken to a playroom, the Romanian children exhibited very similar behaviour patterns:

'When I observed the children in the playroom, they were unaware of each other, fixed on their own activities – barely communicating. Some just sat and seemed bewildered and vacant.' (Reflective Diary, 6 February 2000)

Harlow had concluded that *'no play makes for a very socially disturbed monkey'* (Suomi and Harlow, 1971). We might just as easily conclude that no play makes for a very socially disturbed child.

When Harlow's infants reached physiological maturity they were *'incompetent in virtually every aspect of monkey social activity'* (Suomi and Harlow, 1971). For example, they showed little understanding of social rules or social hierarchy, often preferring to sit in a corner by themselves, and they sometimes engaged in self-harm. In the early months of the playwork project, the Romanian children were showing signs of these disturbing behaviour patterns, as the following extracts illustrate.

'Alexandru still can't keep focused for very long. He started to build bricks on his own today, but after a few moments he was throwing them around again, which is dangerous for the other children. He doesn't seem to be aware of that.' (Reflective Diary, 15 February 2000)

'Elena ... is aware for a few seconds and then looks away. She also smiles a lot but never at the other children. She seldom cries or makes any loud noises. She stares at things endlessly.' (Reflective Diary, 16 February 2000)

'While dressing Carol, I noticed the bruises on his back from him banging the cot. It was awful and covered his whole back. What must these poor kids be thinking when they are tied to the cots each night? Quite a lot of them harm themselves physically.' (Reflective Diary, 28 February 2000)

In contrast to all the evidence of social and physical damage, Harlow found that total isolation had *'little apparent effect on the monkeys' intellectual capabilities'* (Suomi and Harlow, 1971). This was also borne out in our experience of the Romanian children. Virgil, for example, exhibited many disturbing behaviour patterns, such as clutching his feet and rocking at the slightest sign of tension, or refusing to eat unless he was standing up. Nevertheless, the following extract suggests his intellectual capacities remained unimpaired.

'Virgil appears to have made improvements – or maybe he could do these things anyway, but just hasn't been encouraged. He sat with Edit for a few hours and learnt some colours and numbers. He can concentrate for a long time, so he really absorbs what he hears ... It's also excellent how fluent his vocabulary is, considering that last Dec / Jan he couldn't say a word.' (Reflective Diary, 15 February 2000)

As a general rule however, Harlow showed that isolation had a severely damaging impact on an infant monkey's chances of maturing into a stable, functioning adult. Harlow and his collaborators suggested that play, or the absence of it, was an absolutely critical factor in this process. Only provide a little play during the developing years and the ill effects of isolation appear to be negated. The final sentence of their 1971 article is particularly relevant to our work.

'Then pity the monkeys who are not permitted to play, and pray that all children will always be allowed to play.' (Suomi and Harlow, 1971)

Conclusions

Thus far we have presented a fairly shocking picture of abuse and neglect and its appalling consequences. The Romanian children with whom we worked had not been able to play. The results were clearly catastrophic, and might have been thought irreversible. However, our study, echoing Harlow's findings, showed that recovery was still possible even for these severely deprived children.

The following extract was written towards the end of Sophie's first period of working at the hospital. Considering these were the same children who had been tied to their cots, rocking and staring into space only a few months previously, it illustrates the vast change that had taken place in a very short period of time.

'The thing I'm going to miss most of all is coming into the room in the morning. Sometimes Carol or Ion are still sleeping, and it's lovely to be there when they open their eyes. When we open the door there are lots of shouts of happiness and excitement, jumping up and down in their cots. The noise only starts when we open the door, or when they see us through the window – they are so quiet before that. The first thing I do is go around saying good morning to each one and untie them from their cots and get them on the floor. There are lots of morning cuddles.' (Reflective Diary, 29 March 2000)

In less than a year, these chronically abused and neglected children made the sort of progress that many experts assumed would be impossible. During the period of the research study, the only change in the children's life experience was the playwork project. Therefore, it is sensible to ask what it is about playwork that has contributed to these changes. Clearly the children's learning and development resulted substantially from the playworkers' ability to create an enriched play environment that was substantially supportive of the play process. The playworkers' use of negative capability, their suspension of judgment and prejudice, coupled with a determination to take each child's agenda as their own starting point, helped to create a good quality playwork environment – in other words, an environment that offered adaptability to the children, and so encouraged the compound flexibility process.

Through their empathy and their ability to interpret the children's play cues effectively, the playworkers were able to create strong trusting relationships, which in turn helped to enhance the children's self-esteem. If such approaches were applied in a typical playwork setting in the UK we would expect children to learn and develop naturally. The remarkable thing about our experience in Romania was that this straightforward playwork approach appeared to work just as effectively with some of the most play-deprived children in the world.

Editor's comment:

Negative capability revisited

If we can accept such case studies from the world outside the laboratory as legitimate evidence, then accounts like Brown and Webb's raise questions over the claim that early damage is tantamount to irreversible. This in turn raises questions over the current insistence that early intervention is crucial – especially where that insistence goes hand in hand with cuts to funding of other programmes working with vulnerable individuals in later life, in the apparent belief that the crucial stages for intervention have been missed, and it is now too late.

The theme of the liberating nature of play – the space for 'negative capability' as Brown and Webb call it - is something we will find in many areas. However, creating or fostering negative capability is not the same as doing nothing. On the contrary, an awareness of the importance of a safe space to grow into puts still more emphasis on the need to find the practical techniques and processes that can foster this crucial potential.

The practice example that follows looks further at the nature of play. It records a focus-group discussion with a group of early years practitioners, three former colleagues, with considerable experience of working with babies, young children and their families, and practiced in supporting the play of these children. They argue that 'listening' to children is a necessary component at the heart of successful work with children and families, and here they describe the innovation in approach that allowed them to turn playwork into a dynamic, integrative and healing experience, for their children and their families.

They were asked to consider two questions.

1. Is there something special about playwork that helps when working with traumatised or neglected kids, and if so, what is it?
2. Do you find something in what playwork has or does that you can see in other areas of life too?

They were then left to talk about whatever they chose.

Chapter 6
Playing with freedom

Nikki Mellor

The three of us worked together in an Early Years Centre in Islington in the late 90s and early 2000s. The story we want to tell is what happened when we introduced profile books at the centre.

At the Early Years Centre, the profile book was a blank book that was filled by the child, the practitioners, and by the family with anything and everything that speaks about that child's life and experiences.

They ended up being very powerful for the children themselves, but they were also incredibly useful in enabling parents and families to talk openly about things that had happened in their lives. For some they became a way to deal not just with things in the present, but things in the past, allowing people to look at them again and cope with them better. Because this was a very flexible vehicle it worked for both child and family alike; it brought them together, and us more together with them. It helped to integrate the centre, and our work, into the lives of these families.

Early years centres and profile books

This was a community day nursery and so it was open to everybody in the area but we did have six places officially designated for children with a range of complex needs. About one-third or one-quarter of parents had been referred or encouraged to bring their children by health visitors or social workers. Many of them had something or other in their past, some issue. There were lots of examples of past traumatic events in the family, maybe going back many years: some were refugees, for example, and a lot came from quite deprived backgrounds.

These children were very young, from as young as four months up to five years. When you are working with kids so young, you just can't separate the child and the parent; you are working with the whole family. The children might be with us between six to 10 hours a day, and for most children it was the first time they had been away from their parents for any length of time, so we really were a big part of their lives.

These children are very young and exploring the world for the first time, taking their first steps, for example, while the mother is not there. The parents had to leave the child with us, and they needed to be able to trust us. So we had to work out how to do this. How do we offer something that really helps and supports families to understand what is happening here, what we are doing and how they can be part of it? How do we give them a voice?

We started using profile books simply as a record of the children's progress and development – their learning journey, as it is called. We had a keyworker system – a key person for each child – and every key person made up a book for each of their key children to be used as a record of what the child was doing and learning. In the book we could put pictures they had made, or photos that we took. The book is then full of visual memories for children who can't read yet. We could also write in for them some of their own words – or utterances, because many of the youngest children were not using words properly yet, or not full sentences.

The profile books really put the child at the centre of everything that happens there. In them, they see themselves and their lives mirrored – quite literally sometimes, because we would often put in pictures of them and small mirrors. The whole thing was really empowering. It was really about giving a voice to the children, enabling them to make something that is shared and that communicates.

Then, by putting the child at the heart, they can see the continuity in their life and in their learning. For example, during transitions such as when they go to first visit a new school, we might put in a photo of the school, and a picture of the new key person; something to ease the process. The child can then look back, and think, 'Well, I dealt with that change; I can deal with others'. They can reflect on their own learning journey and learn from that reflection.

You have really got to appreciate that everyday things can be traumatic for children, and they need to know that we appreciate how they feel. We don't want them to grow up thinking being hurt or frightened is OK, not just for them but also other people.

It might not be a big thing therefore, or it might not seem so to us. For one child it might concern a fear of balloons, or of medicine, and they might want the world to know they are afraid of these things. Putting it in the book reassures them that adults know about it, and know how they feel.

I remember an 18-month-old boy who seemed to be quite independent and he rarely talked. I wasn't his key person. However, I remember one day he arrived at nursery with a cut on his thumb covered with a plaster. It was so important to him that he spent the first hour of the day searching out every adult he could find to show them his finger, take off the plaster and explain how his injury had come about. Of course, the adults were all very sympathetic and helped him find the words to describe what had happened.

He played outside and the plaster quickly came off, and so I asked him if I should put it into his profile book. He agreed, and wanted a photo of the cut on his thumb, which he then stuck it into his book. He told me what to write, '*J hurt finger, blood, plaster*'. He then proceeded to show the page to other children and adults, and by the end of the afternoon he wanted us to add, '*better now*'.

The ability of children to also help each other via profile books is enormous. When a child was upset, for example, another child might go and give them their book – it was as if they were saying, 'Here, you'll be needing this'.

Some children slept with their books, and one new child would only sleep in the nursery if she had her book next to her on a bookshelf open at the page where there was a picture of her mother.

There is an important message in there about diversity. Even for those who can't speak or write for themselves the book says, 'This is me, this is who I am, this is what I do, what I can do. This is what I don't like, and what I do like.' We are all individuals after all. You are not special because you are different, you are special because you are you.

The role of keyworkers

Every child had a key person who was their advocate within the centre and who became a special person for that child. They gave each child the opportunity to develop a close relationship with one or sometimes two particular people. Within the security of this relationship the child would go on to develop relationships with other adults and children, but the key person remained special for them (Elfer, 2003). (It is now a statutory obligation for all children in early years provision to have a key person.)

The key people also build close relationships with the parents so you can keep them up to date about what their child is doing, what they are learning and who their friends are. Their child's time at the centre is literally an open book, and even very young children can have long detailed conversations about what happens in the centre with their parents using the visual clues contained in the books.

At one point we visited another nursery at which they were doing something more – including the parents' voices in their profile books. While it was just us practitioners and the children who wrote in the books, we hadn't encouraged parents to join in. Straightaway we said, *'We've got to do that'*, and so we used their approach to enhance what we were doing.

There was the element of having time for reflection. One thing that really made it work, and what gave it strength, was our ability to learn how to enable it to happen. That was the real foundation – our ability to make mistakes and learn from them. It was the talking together. It was about investing the time to revisit what we were doing, discussing, supporting new staff, bringing others up to speed. That is how you really realise what you do – when you are describing it to someone else.

It didn't work with everyone though – not only did some parents not quite get it, but sometimes the key person didn't either. It wouldn't have worked therefore if we weren't a team and if there wasn't someone else around to support them.

Another reason we could make it work was that we made people feel safe; it was all born out of a trusting relationship. I have seen many profile books since then, learning journeys and so on in other settings, but we also created an ethos, so that people really knew we were rooting for their child. We all felt safe within this relationship of trust and we had the whole environment working to make the relationships work.

Involving the parents

The centre was small by some standards – with 70 families. That is still quite a lot, but the space we had was focused, so we had the quality and the intimacy to make it feel safe and secure. You could get to know everybody, and they knew each other. That really helped. The layout of rooms was important here, too – having the flexibility to change the way we used the space, even change the space we had available to us, just by propping a door open, moving a table outside, making a ladder on the climbing frame lower for the child who had just decided to try to climb, putting out a favourite book for a new child. Together we set up the centre as an enabling environment for the children.

What really mattered most was having the time and opportunity to discuss things with a parent, and to go a little bit deeper in order to engage them. We introduced the books and explained them to the parent, quickly realising that we needed to help them and encourage them, so they could get involved. We therefore organised workshops for parents so that they could use the profile book with their child at the workshop. They really took to it, and they would bring in their own pictures of home and family.

I thought we were good with parents. Of course, we could always do better, but until the profile books came along we didn't really know how to. That's what focused and crystallised it, and brought it all out of us. The books gave us the confidence and a vehicle to talk about what we thought our work really was, and how we helped their child learn. It gave the parents the chance to share in this and teach us about the individuality of their child. It built a partnership with the child at the heart.

It was then that we realised that a parent could also make up their own profile book, for themselves – not just for the child – and some of them did. It was quite organic; it just evolved. We couldn't stop it happening!

One example sticks in my mind particularly. X was the mother of a child in care who was living with a grandparent, but she was able to come to the centre to discuss what her child was doing and be involved. Because we had the profile books she could see what we were doing and what her child was doing. Now they have something to look back on in the family.

One day, X talked to us about her child being in care. With the help of the profile books she could feel safe enough to talk about things.

Another woman had been in a car accident in which her child had suffered a brain injury. She hadn't ever wanted to talk about it and she had to keep it at a distance. Putting it in the book, however, somehow kept it at a safe distance but still kept it in the world. *'Then I won't have to block it out,'* she said, *'because it* ***is*** *part of his life and it needs to be there'*. I felt very privileged that parents were talking to me about things that were distressing, and I knew that this was going to be huge for the family.

There was another incident where there had been a flood in a child's grandmother's flat. The grandmother brought in the sodden book to see if I could help dry it out. It's amazing to think that, despite the flooded flat, retrieving the book was still so important.

Children with complex needs

The children with complex needs were the ones who used the profile books most, but they weren't singled out in any way – every child had a profile book. The difference wasn't in the kids, therefore, but in the way we worked with them. Very often with children with complex needs people tend to focus on what the child doesn't do, but their profile book focuses on what they can do and what new things they are learning every day. One parent of a child with complex special needs cried when she first saw her child's profile book. *'This is the first time someone has told me what my child can do,'* she said, *'Everyone else seems more interested in what he can't do.'*

We had a 'Teens and Toddlers' project with kids from the local secondary school who had been excluded. They would send a group down to the nursery and they would play with the children for a couple of weeks, and then perhaps they would be partnered up with one child in particular. We backed off and let them learn together.

Sometimes it could bring out the best in these troubled kids because they felt respected, listened to. They also had a mini profile books of their own during the project. For some of them it was a clear realisation about the needs of these little children, but it also got them thinking about their own lives. That situation has a lot of potential.

The nature of play and the development of the child

It is vital to let children play, to revisit and reflect on their ideas. Our work is all about creating a safe environment for them to experiment and try out their ideas in all areas of their learning, be it emotional, social or intellectual. It is also essential to observe children closely and support them in their investigations. If, for example, we find one pre-verbal child relates to the world by throwing things around, you throw things with them – safely, of course, but you throw. Others will hang back and just watch, and so you hang back too and watch with them. They are still playing and they are learning, just as we all are.

Communicating with the children, and your relationships with them, are like scaffolding. It is said that children can do things with an adult they feel safe and confident with that they could not yet do alone. We see that every day.

When adults sing, talk with friends, play or listen to music, go for a walk, give support to friends in hard times or cook a special meal, they are playing too. Investigating and learning while playing. In early years work, we are workers who are given the permission to work with play. So we are playing too – we too are given the freedom to give them that freedom.

Looking forward

We have to hope, if early intervention becomes the next big thing to prevent social exclusion and disadvantage, that we get to keep a space for this creativity. It would be a shame to see a curriculum enforced, with milestones, targets we have to get them to achieve. Kids need the freedom to learn, and that's what we have to give them. That, and believing that they matter.

All children have a right to a childhood with the kind of rich, exciting fun experiences that enable them to see themselves as proficient learners and good people. That's what childhood should be about, not getting ready to be older and being taught to fit into a system that does not value individuality or recognise potential. If nothing else, profile books give children the opportunity to remember there was a time when they were loved and appreciated because they are loveable and worth the effort.

I can't imagine working without profile books now. I have to sometimes, working in other places, but I can't understand for the life of me why people would not do this.

Editor's comment: A vehicle for self-possession

These workers describe profile books as a vehicle, not a technique. It is perhaps worth dwelling on the distinction. A technique is a tool to do some specific thing, and the test of a good tool – as of the tool user – is whether it gets you the results you wanted. A vehicle is a way to carry something else, and what that something is may be entirely individual. It may also be entirely new.

This is a theme that we will find again and again in the case studies of practice.

These playworkers describe the relationships they created and the safe 'enabling' environment as 'a scaffolding' that allows the children to grow in their own way. The role of the whole environment and the use of the environment to create a non-directive and liberating space is another theme that will reappear.

So consistent is this thread in the accounts that follow that it suggests that for those who have experienced trauma, neglect and rejection in their lives, it is particularly important that future experiences, and especially those with care-givers and figures of power and authority, are able to give them the emotional space to reclaim their own self-control.

In the next two examples we can see the same issues in the context now of adolescents. This is not to say, of course, that the children and young people here have personality disorders, or even that they are necessarily on the way to lives of complex and compound trauma. However many, if not most, have experiences of abuse or neglect, and many are showing signs of the complex and conflicted relationships that, if unchecked and mismanaged, may become embedded and self-perpetuating ways of relating to the world. These services, we argue, are preventive, and it is from prevention, just as much as from cure, that we can learn the most helpful lessons.

Chapter 7
For argument's sake

Will Smith and Jessica Dix

Debate Mate is a relatively new educational charity that runs after-school debating clubs in schools in areas of high child poverty. It uses debating to build children's confidence and self-esteem, improve their academic achievement and develop communication, higher order thinking and interpersonal skills in a constructive, positive and safe environment. Learning to debate empowers young people, giving them a voice and the skills needed to engage with the issues that affect them, and helps them to find solutions.

During debates, pupils have to critically respond to what is said by other participants, developing their listening skills in a way that activities such as public speaking do not. Indeed, listening skills are the skills that pupils and teachers regularly report to have improved the most. In particular, the rules of debating ensure that all have an equal say – debates are not dominated by louder and more confident pupils, and these pupils learn the importance of listening, while those that often do not play a commanding role in class discussions are given the opportunity to make valuable contributions.

Debates have two teams, a proposition and an opposition. Each team must work as a unit in order to be successful. Pupils must come up with arguments, assess and prioritise their ideas and divide them out among the speakers in a limited amount of time before the debate begins (usually 20 minutes). As each team has at least four pupils it is crucial that they prepare effectively, with different pupils taking different roles. In particular, they must manage their preparation time as a team effectively, ensuring nobody plays too big or too small a role, while some take on leadership roles directing the group's discussion.

Debating requires young people to consider arguments for positions and opinions they themselves do not hold. They are therefore pushed to question the arguments that they then put forwards, and develop them to be as persuasive as possible. Learners must react to the arguments of others, and respond to them in a critical way, making this an ideal vehicle for developing critical thinking skills.

Debating also engages young people with issues that they might not normally have encountered. In most debates pupils are identifying possible solutions to problems and presenting a case for or against those solutions. Vitally, debating develops the skills necessary to effectively approach and engage with issues of concern.

Perhaps most important, however, is the fact that debating's formal structures provide a channel for non-violent expression. Behavioural difficulties can often be traced to an inability to verbalise and articulate emotion, and debating enables young people to be able to do exactly this. Furthermore, these formal structures and the turn-taking nature of debating allow energy and conflict to be channelled positively.

At the heart of the Debate Mate programme is self and peer assessment. In order to progress, pupils are encouraged to reflect on their performance and set themselves targets for improvement. Crucially, pupils assess each other through judging the debates they take part in, offering detailed feedback to their peers after each debate.

Debate Mate recruits successful and inspiring university students to run its debate clubs – the programme is delivered almost exclusively by 18 to 23-year-olds. This ensures that Debate Mate mentors can also act as role models for young people who are unlikely to find role models elsewhere. Often for the first time in their lives participants in Debate Mate's programmes begin to make plans for university and for their future careers. It really does inspire them.

The programme began in 2009, and it is perhaps too soon to expect to see the long-term impact through formal research. This story can as yet only be told via a few case studies, but there is already significant anecdotal evidence of Debate Mate's positive impact upon those who were otherwise likely to be excluded, or those with behavioural problems.

Debate Mate's programmes work because young people almost unanimously enjoy debating: 99% of participants in the 2010–2011 programme said that they enjoyed participating in the programme. Nearly 2500 young people currently take part in Debate Mate clubs each week, now operating in London, Birmingham, Manchester and Bristol.

Here are just a few examples of those the programme has helped. (Note that all the young people named here were happy to have their own names used.)

Case studies

Lewis, at the age of 14, was a very able pupil, yet found himself unchallenged. Becoming disaffected, he often found himself in detention.

He was exposed to debating through Debate Mate's precursor, the London Debate Challenge (2002–2003). The skills he learnt gave him a passion for debating and a purpose. He was made captain of the England Schools' Debating Team.

Through debating Lewis entered Oxford University, became the first black president of the Oxford Student Union and he is now the World Debating Champion and a trainee at Slaughter & May, a leading international law firm.

'Debate Mate gives young people one of the most useful skills possible, that is, the ability to speak and debate. I would not be where I am without debating. It turned my life around.'

Sendeniz, aged 15, was disengaged with school and was marked as a possible dropout. Her lack of interest in education led to low self-esteem and truancy.

Debate Mate helped build her confidence and find her place in school as a leader. Through us she recognised the importance of school and was inspired to learn about the world around her, leading to improved attendance and grades.

She helped run Debate Mate in her old school and now plans to set up a debating club at her new college.

'The most significant thing Debate Mate has done is encourage me to attend school. I wasn't allowed to go to a session once because I was skipping school. I cried for the hour it was going on.'

15-year-old **Dangelo** was a troubled student. Following expulsion from two schools he saw himself as at risk of engaging in gang culture and violent behaviour.

Debate Mate gave him an opportunity to succeed where the traditional educational process had failed him. Through debating he was able to express himself through a competitive yet ultimately intellectual activity. Developing sophisticated verbal skills, Dangelo found a voice, learning to resolve conflict without resorting to violence.

He is now head boy at his school, and aims to study law or medicine. He was also the subject of a newspaper article, 'The boy who refused to riot' (Trew, *Evening Standard*, 5 September 2011) in which he explained how Debate Mate turned his life around.

'If I hadn't done Debate Mate I would have been a part of the riots, but I've changed my outlook ... I've realised you're not tied to what you were born into.'

Editor's comment:

The great debate

While the majority of participants are between 12 and 15 years old, Debate Mate has run successful programmes with nine to 11-year-olds and also with socially excluded 18 to 24-year-olds, for example, in partnership with Kids Company and The Urban Academy. In the following chapter, one of the Kids Company staff describes the effectiveness of debate, as a skill and a technique for engaging their disaffected youngsters.

Kids Company is another example of an exceptionally dynamic and innovative organisation that is rapidly growing, and it bases much of its work on attachment theory. They have gone on to develop research programmes focused on an understanding of the behaviour of traumatised children in the light of contemporary neuroscience. Their slogan, to stress the importance of a slow, steady rebuilding of children's emotional lives, is *'One neuron at a time'*.

A simple example may serve to illustrate the pervasiveness of psychotherapeutic thinking in their work. At the Urban Academy, which specialises in education for youngsters excluded from mainstream schools, all the teaching staff have regular supervision with trained counsellors. The academy also has security staff, in the event of disruptive behaviour. The security staff, who by virtue of their role are often at the heart of conflict, also receive supervision from the same counsellors.

Chapter 8
Debating at The Urban Academy

Chiedza Chashe Preddie

Having met Margaret McCabe, we were immediately smitten by what Debate Mate had to offer: the development of communication, teamwork and leadership skills for our students. We invited them to work with us and a few short months later we had our own Debate Mate class set up, with a dedicated teacher coming to lead us on a Friday afternoon at The urban Academy – the post-16 educational centre of Kids Company.

The sessions were lively and fun-filled, and they gave the students a space to express their views, to enhance their interpersonal skills and, especially, to be heard. Basic debating skills were learnt and were deeply embedded. It was an absolute joy to see unsure, reticent young people stand up and 'state their case' with confidence. Even the most confident of speakers learned how to hone their natural skills of articulation and persuasion.

As the Debate Mate programme was designed with secondary school age students in mind, we adapted it to fit our more mature and streetwise group of teens and young adults. The topics under debate ranged from 'This house believes that the best way to dump somebody is by Facebook' to 'This house believes that Black History Month is a perfect example of institutional racism'. Class numbers rocketed from an average of five students to over 17. This was assisted by making the debates open to all – students from other classes and staff alike. Debating lessons were brought out of the classroom and into the more public setting of the dining room.

The most popular and well attended debate was the one held in the summer of 2010. The motion was 'This house believes that prejudice and discrimination is still rife within the police force'. Representatives from the local police force were invited to form the opposition team. The all-male student debaters were most impressive, displaying superb debating and communication skills, detailed knowledge and understanding of the law and their rights. The even-handed way in which they dealt with such a potentially controversial topic was remarkable, and the cause for much discussion several days later. The students who formed the proposition team won by a clear majority of votes and were a credit not only to The Urban Academy or Kids Company but, ultimately, they were a credit to themselves.

Adapting the topics in this way to our kids' real life concerns helped ensure the success of the programme, so that the debates continued, with energy and vigour, after the Debate Mate teacher left. It pleases us to say that, after a year's absence, our debating lesson is back on the timetable at The Urban Academy and will be used as the main vehicle for delivering the Open College Network's Prejudice and Discrimination accredited course.

The riots of Summer 2011 have shown that it is even more essential for our young people to be able to articulate, express, personally develop their interpersonal and intrapersonal skills in these uncertain times.

Editor's comment: The future in the present

Debate is a technique that, like the introduction of profile books, is best seen as a vehicle for self-expression – in this case, one better suited to older children and teenagers. Here, peer engagement and peer feedback are a key part of the formal structure – which is, again, peculiarly appropriate for the development of social skills in later childhood and adolescence.

The next example continues to explore lessons in innovation when working with young people at risk of exclusion, again demonstrating the importance of encouraging self-expression and the role of peer relationships.

In the following edited extract from an interview, Jean Templeton describes the thinking behind the development of St Basils' philosophy and services. St Basils works with young people who are homeless or at risk, providing services ranging from prevention and early intervention work, through to crisis intervention and stabilisation, resettlement and re-integration. St Basils engages young people at all points along the pathway, whether they are 'at risk' or gaining confidence and skills, or moving on to independent living. Importantly, the pathway is based on the young person's own natural journey towards autonomy.

St Basils have committed themselves to becoming a more 'psychologically informed environment'. However, this is not an account of one single coherent environment, but a disparate yet carefully and flexibly integrated network of services and resources, which move around the young person. This is highly significant as it reflects not just the multiplicity of ways in which youth at risk may find themselves in need of St Basils' services, and the range of their needs, but also the multiple possibilities that are typical of youthful exploration.

Here we explore some of the issues that that ambition throws up.

Chapter 9
Turmoil and transition:
St Basils

Jean Templeton, CEO

Our core client group is young people aged between 16 and 25, although we also do schools outreach work, mentoring and awareness, which often start earlier. Family mediation can also refer younger people for early intervention. This work is mainly with school years 10 or 11, but we also work with youth clubs and so we can start to engage young people earlier. The majority of our work, however, is increasingly with 16 to 21-year-olds. We don't work with people past the age of 25. This is deliberate, not just a consequence of limited funding or contracts, as it gives us a horizon to aim for, in time.

This is important because in our model we are not solely concerned with the immediate problem, but are keen to respond to the presenting problem in the context of where the young person wishes to be in the longer term. We use what is called a 'logic chain' model. There are many variations around but the one we use is originally based on the Canadian Government's approach to problem solving, that is, first we look at the young person's longer-term goals, then work back from these to ensure that progress made is in the service of those goals both in the medium term and while addressing their immediate needs. That reversal of the usual sequence is central in order that any intervention can contribute to the longer-term goal and not derail this inadvertently.

For example, take homelessness. We know that young people may believe that in order to secure assistance they will have to say that they have nowhere at all to sleep and no-one who will have them. However, if you simply respond to that, if you make that the issue that your service is all about, then the young person will be placed in possibly unsuitable emergency accommodation, and there they will simply languish for a while. If the problem to be addressed is merely seen as finding a bed, all efforts will be focused on getting accommodation.

However, we also know that that is very likely to be poor quality accommodation, probably in an unhelpful area. Once placed there, they may find it difficult to move out, and if they don't just abandon the tenancy and leave, the impact on the young person's self-esteem, and their ambitions for their lives, may be lasting. Therefore, if you always deal first with the immediate presenting need, and all your strategies and interventions are then geared to that, if you only deal with people at the point of crisis, then you will always get more crises. Crisis becomes the currency you are dealing in.

The whole idea of the logic approach is to maintain a focus on the future, on their ambitions and their goals, and then focus on what they need to do and what help they need from us in order to progress towards achieving them. We therefore ask the young person where they see themselves in five years' time, and work with them to identify what they need to do in order to achieve their goal. Not all young people have thought about this and so the process is slower. The initial assessment will start to develop the conversation, the immediate needs can be met, the young person assisted to settle, and the discussion continues about their ambitions and aspirations.

While young people don't always recognise the questions initially, on building trust with their support worker they will start to discuss the areas in which they would like to progress. This may involve improving relationships with their family, or it may concern education and training. It may be learning to read or tackling their drug or alcohol dependency. When you ask what they want to achieve, there is always ambition there.

If one is a violent offender, for example, it may be that the goal is to assist the young person to deal with conflict without resorting to violence. This will mean that future relationships are not blighted by violence and that any children they have will not witness violence as a means of resolving disagreements.

Of course, this is not to ignore the presenting problems, the current crisis. We also have to deal with those. We aim to reduce the number of young people who come to us in crisis by our prevention work and increase early intervention and planned entry. However, we always stress that this is just for now, and that even what we do immediately must be informed by what the young person would like to do in the future and what they need to get there. On that basis, we draw up needs assessments and action plans. Looking far enough ahead may quite often change their initial response.

It is not, therefore, just about needs, and it is not about creating dependency. Everything we do is about reinforcing ambition and moving towards independence. Essentially, St Basils is about fuelling aspiration and building capability. If we want to raise the young person's aspirations we must support them to believe in themselves as well as help them develop practical skills. We encourage them to make safe, informed judgments, and to have the confidence to make them. We therefore have a Life Skills Programme, which is accredited with the Open College Network, and we give employability training, which includes writing a CV and preparing for interviews etc.

All the training we provide is fully recognised, with qualifications scored and accredited to NVQ Levels One and Two. Every year we have a graduation ceremony for which we hire caps and gowns. The young people are encouraged to invite their family – their mums and dads, but also siblings, whoever the young person feels close to, whoever they want to invite, to share their success. Again, that is about reinforcing – for many, this may be the first time for years that the family have seen them doing something good.

There are other ways to enhance people's self-esteem. One is to really listen to what they are saying, and so we have our Youth Advisory Board – 15 young people who are elected by their peers and trained for the role. It is all about influencing the environment you are in and it is seen as prestigious within our community.

We also facilitate the National Youth Reference Group, which is funded by the Department of Communities and Local Government (CLG) to advise government and local government on tackling youth homelessness. Young people from around the country have joined the National Youth Reference Group, where they receive training and support to identify what has worked for them and what is not effective. They have developed a website and various guides to codify their experiences and provide guidance to policy makers and service providers on how to tackle and prevent homelessness in the young population.

Over the years, St Basils grew organically, adding in new services and ventures as the need and opportunity arose. We then decided that it was time for a review, to see where we are going and how it all hangs together. What are our main outcomes, we asked ourselves, and how can we be more intentional about making that happen? How can we sustain and even intensify what we do? We looked at our previous organic growth and we remodelled.

For example, we have now restructured and we have formally separated our housing service from the support service, so that support workers can follow the individual wherever they are living. This is in line with recent Supporting People policy, but it was not just for contractual reasons – young people have said they want the continuity of trust and relationship.

This also means that we can reflect more realistically the mainstream world of housing, with landlords and rent and dealing with neighbours – having responsibilities, taking the consequences. All our accommodation is high quality. And it is all short term – young people stay a maximum of two years, usually much less – before going on to other landlords. We are clearer now about the two highly skilled roles of housing management and support, and where our own responsibility starts and ends, and we will go as far as eviction if we have to. Now, however, if we do, we can continue the support.

In fact, we liken this to being in higher education. If you think about it, those who are reasonably successful in education will then find their lives, challenges and social learning mapped out for them in a fairly structured way. They usually start out in halls of residence, with others all around them, other students, staff and so on. They can experiment a lot with new freedoms, but there are people around to make sure they don't do anything too daft. In the second year they might move out to a shared flat, and then move again in the third year.

They learn to make some compromises – a slightly less attractive flat, for example, as a trade-off for lower rent, or a less attractive area to be closer to college. They never had these choices when they lived at home, and so they are learning these skills as well as getting marketable qualifications. These are all staged transitions – all purposeful, moving the person on and up towards your goals. It is a three-year rite of passage.

Conversely, for those not successful in the education system, there is none of that. No pathway, no integration, no eased transitions. At St Basils we try to integrate education and training support with accommodation, to build in those stages and rites of passage. It is quite age appropriate to be moving through housing. People should not have to be either homeless or successful in higher education to get this structure to grow within.

First and foremost we are a youth agency who use housing as the medium to work with young people; that is at the heart of everything we do. Because we work with young people only, we can place the young person at the centre. However, we are also a 'connector' service: we link into all other related strategies and services, working with partners who can support young people. 87% of our youngsters are not in education, employment or training, and many have been involved with the criminal justice system. 25% are or were 'looked after' by Social Services, and over 40% have no qualifications.

So if we can engage other services, so much the better. We tell them, we are a resource for you. We have a captive audience – we have with us some of the most excluded young people in the area, just the ones that you need to reach. So why would you not want to work with us? We help you access that group, and so achieve the goals you are here to achieve.

For example, we became interested in becoming a more psychologically informed environment (PIE) during the initial consultations that led up to the production of the CLG/National Mental Health Development Unit guidance (2010). Our initial response to the CLG guidance was cautious and we were keen not to pathologise young people, feeling that the study related much more to rough sleepers and people with very entrenched problems. How far does it really apply to youth?

However the idea of 'complex trauma' resonated with us, and here the guidance seemed to describe many of the difficulties that we were picking up in our work. We followed up with Dr Nick McGuire from Southampton University and, following lengthy discussion and consideration, we decided to invest in developing St Basils as a PIE, in partnership with Birmingham and Solihull Mental Health Foundation Trust. The trust had launched a consultation (see Youthspace Birmingham at www.youthspace.me/about/about.aspx) on how to develop their mental health services for young people. The response was that they needed to reshape their services to come more from a youth perspective. They now want to deliver services in non-institutional environments, and we can offer the premises for them – so the partnership started.

We have also now agreed extra support for our own staff. A senior clinical psychologist will work with us once a week and we plan to have, for example, 1.5 hours for assisted reflective practice to review cases, and to help us think about what we are doing. We are therefore committing to develop as a PIE – we have the funding, we are developing some baseline indicators, and we will have training for all staff and reflective practice built in, just as the PIE approach suggests.

There are still some dilemmas we need to resolve however. We are not a mental health service, and we don't want to pathologise our young people. We don't want them to see the words 'psychologically informed' and think that means we are a treatment service. If we are training staff to have an understanding of psychological approaches, we still don't need and don't want to *be* psychologists.

We may want to develop as a PIE, but we are not going to be therapists, whether for the young people or the staff. (It is good that people do recognise their own issues, but if they really want to work on their own issues, they do it in their own time.) We do not want to become a therapeutic community (TC) and spend all our time discussing the internal dynamics of the organisation. We do not want St Basils even to be seen as a TC; that would be mis-selling.

It is not even about treatment – we do not have to know about that. It might sometimes help to know something about treatment options and styles – if only because that helps de-mythologise mental health. It is good to have a better understanding of what those services have to offer, a better idea of what *is* within their scope, and what needs they can meet. Having access to information on services, and having them operating here, can prevent people panicking at the idea of mental health problems. If that helps slow down the cascade on interventions and the defensive practice of referral to specialist services, that has got to be good for everyone.

To me, it is much more about understanding young people's adolescent development, and what gets in the way of normal transitions, of familiar patterns of growing up, adolescent turmoil, testing out and so on. Young people without any trauma in their background can still create havoc, test the boundaries and rebel. This is the ordinary and healthy chaos of adolescence.

It is not, therefore, all about clinical psychology – we really need an understanding about normal development and the barriers to it. We need to be better informed about ordinary turmoil, what the pathways for young people are, and then what can derail their development and learning, what the risks are and how to pull things back.

It is good to have an understanding of child and adolescent development in terms of behavioural psychology, attachment and so on. That is about establishing a level of knowledge to inform our practice, to help build their (and our) resilience, so that we do not just get stressed and react if someone's behaviour is provoking or disruptive. It enables us to hit the pause button and take a step backwards. Don't just do something – stand there.

The key question for us is recognising how much of this behaviour is ordinary adolescence, and how much stems from other, deeper problems that need addressing.

This is because it is not our background and we need to know what we are doing and what psychology is the most appropriate for us. We are weakest is in understanding where ordinary psychological development and maturation can go awry, and disrupt or disturb natural development. Violent abuse and separation traumas for example; for some, it is these things that have contributed to homelessness.

In fact, the young people in the National Youth Reference Group may talk from a quite theoretically uninformed position, but still they speak from a very real psychological awareness:

'If we behave badly, sometimes things have happened to us that change our personalities and make us behave really badly. That doesn't mean that we are bad people ... You may have to understand that if we do act up, play stuff out, it's because of something else that's happened...'

Then there are those who have come through the care system, some of them with very complex needs. However, there seems to be many factors contributing to a higher needs profile among the young people we are seeing. Since the Southwark ruling (a legal judgment over the responsibilities of local authorities' Social Services), we are seeing a much higher proportion of 16 and 17-year-olds. We have also seen changes in housing benefit regulations, which will mean that people under 35 cannot get rent for an individual flat. Also, since the removal of the Supporting People funding 'ring-fence', our funding is not so anchored in one funding source's set of outcomes and measures; we can ask new questions.

It changes all the time – changes in the law or benefits mean changes in the profile of our young people. There is constant tectonic plate movement, and we have to be able to respond.

However, even so – even where there is plenty of evidence for emotional disturbance – we hope that, if we are better psychologically informed, we will be more aware of some of the underlying problems, and therefore have better and more effective responses in how we work.

We now really need to think about the implications for the way we operate. There is that element of triage – it is really important that we do not presuppose any level of need, or level of readiness. But then we need to decide how to deal with that range of needs – and the readiness – because sometimes we have to wait, just be there, build up some trust until they are ready to let us in.

Are the same approaches applicable to all? If we have more young people with intensive needs, at what point do we need something more specialist? Do you need specialist interventions at all, or do you attempt to normalise and accommodate them all in standard services? What do we do about behaviour in communal settings, where others are affected? These are the ongoing dilemmas – to be consistent, or to be flexible; to be person-centred, or to be fair.

These are the kinds of questions we need to think about, so that we can respond better. This is what becoming a PIE means, for us.

Editor's comment:
Future-paced work

The big questions for young people are who am I, and what will I be?

When working with young people, these issues have to be constantly to the fore. If we instead define their lives in terms of their immediate presenting issues, and let this immediate need define their relations with us, through eligibility criteria and through tightly measured 'performance outcomes', we are in danger of fixing their sense of who they *are* in who they *were*.

By contrast, St Basils aims to see the young person as a whole, with their future as much a part of who they are now as their past is. The key to the St Basils approach is that this is essentially future-paced work, and that is especially right for teenagers. That is to say, it is age-appropriate, because teenagers live all their lives in the hectic trajectory towards becoming an adult, and in the inevitable, creative uncertainty about what the future holds and how they can make it work.

This work is therefore not solely, or even primarily, about understanding individual psychology. It is as much about understanding the nature and the meaning of youth in the modern age. This is already a highly sociologically informed environment – informed not so much about psychology, and psychopathology, as about ordinary adolescent development, and understanding where this individual is in their lives. The question St Basils is now addressing is how to get the best of both worlds.

How much does their young people's recovery need to focus on the future and their ambitions? But this is a question that does not simply apply to young people.

St Basils' questions for their own service involve questioning the role of psychology as well as questioning their own practice. What do we actually mean by psychology? Is it a question of formal research or a clinical specialism? Or is it more about mind-mindedness and emotional intelligence?

Perhaps what matters most is taking these questions seriously, and taking the time to think it all through as a team. That takes time and commitment, which involves convincing your service's commissioners that it is time they should be funding.

Note here, too, the St Basils team's wariness of the suggestion that they might become a 'therapeutic community'. Part of the intention in proposing the term 'psychologically informed' was to get away from the therapeutic community model – the need to open a second front. There has to be more than one good game in town. This is an issue we will return to in the concluding section.

Meanwhile, there is plenty to suggest that staff training is best when done *in situ* in order for the learning to lead to lasting change. Experiences that you have gone through together, as a group, you can then use together. This enhances the aspect of group reinforcement of new learning, and that in turn enables the ongoing and pervasive reflectiveness that leads to change. Reflective practice that doesn't lead to an enhanced service is just an improving technique, not an improved outcome.

Editor's comment: Crime and disorder

In Chapter 1: Everybody's problem, Rex Haigh has already commented on the extent of PD in the prison population, and it is tempting to assume that here, if anywhere, we will find those hardened criminal types that the notion of an antisocial personality disorder conjures up. It would be foolish to deny that there are such characters, but how typical they are of the prison population is harder to say, and how they got to be that way, and what can be done, are different questions entirely.

Many studies of the mental health needs found in the prison population suggest that there are mental health difficulties of all kinds, and that in remand prisons, with younger prisoners and with women, we find particular difficulties.

Until such time as an issue is thoroughly and systematically researched, anecdotal information may often be the only information that we have to go on, to build up our picture of what may be happening. This does not make anecdotal information untrue, merely unreliable. However, anecdotal evidence – especially from a reliable source, combined often with circumstantial evidence, and with a certain amount of deduction from what we *do* know – may be the precursor or impetus for studying something on a sufficiently large scale for there to be real evidence, one way or another.

The following chapter is a reflection upon a discussion between two colleagues. We place it here in the 'practice' section, on the grounds that the conceptual tools that we use for the clinical assessment of mental health difficulties are themselves a part of essentially social practice – the practice of assessment and diagnosis, taking place in a particular setting, conducted by particular people. The mindset of a professional culture can in itself create a context in which some issues will come to the fore, and others are harder to reach.

Chapter 10

On assessment:

PD typologies and 'learned defiance' in the prison population

Robin Johnson (extract from a presentation at Nottingham Café Scientifique)

This essay records a conversation I personally had some time ago with a former colleague who was at the time contracted to provide psychiatric assessments to the youth remand and young persons' prisons in the local area. My colleague – I will not name her – had found, much as she expected to find, that a significant proportion of the people who were referred to her did indeed have psychiatric problems.

There was a relatively low level of frank psychosis compared to some studies. There was a high incidence of depression and anxiety, and a high incidence of personality disorder (PD). However, what she found striking was that when she came to look beyond the broad category of PD to look at the particular PDs that she was identifying, there was a surprise.

The statistics on mental health in the adult prison population would suggest that it is the 'antisocial' type PD (ASPD) that predominates in the prison population, and this would fit with general expectations of the life course of an ASPD and the high risk of behaving in a way that leads to imprisonment. However, my colleague found that when it came to young offenders specifically:

- roughly one-third of the young prisoners with PD referred to her could be diagnosed as having an ASPD
- roughly one-third could be seen as having a paranoid PD
- roughly one third had an avoidant-dependent PD.

In layman's terms, the paranoid type is the person with a chip on their shoulder who will not back down and the avoidant-dependent is the person who does not like the responsibility for making decisions, and so may be easily led. In each case, it is easy to see how they might be over-represented in youth delinquency, and later in custody. Nevertheless, this apparent disparity between the PD profile in the youth and remand wings, and the profile found in the adult prisons, is certainly interesting. There are a number of possible explanations.

The first is that my colleague was simply wrong and that her clinical judgment was not entirely reliable. Psychiatry is a profession in which disagreement between professionals over the precise formulation of a diagnosis is endemic. It is not a-typical and it casts no real aspersions on her competence to say that another clinician, with another mindset or personality, might have seen something different, or drawn out a different aspect in the personalities of the individual they saw. A clinical assessment, however rigorous, is still a dialogue, after all, between two people. So there is always the possibility of some degree of bias in the way my colleague interpreted the data of interviews.

Another possible source of skew to make her clinical findings an unreliable guide could be that the prison staff, knowing her interest in psychiatric problems over and beyond the narrow range of psychoses etc, might have referred to her a wider range of youngsters than they may otherwise have done, and that therefore the people that she was seeing reflects a skew in the referral mechanism, and the cohort that she saw, in that prison. However, that in itself would still suggest something about the wider range of people in that population that it was possible to refer to her (because they were there), but who are not typically referred to other clinicians. It would mean that there is some social process of filtering referrals, and this in turn would mean that clinical assessments cannot be the only reliable measure of the mental health of the prison population, and survey approaches, for example, might be important.

A third possibility is that it is in fact the case that in youth and remand wings you get a wider range of PDs than you might find in adult prisons. These non-antisocial individuals are perhaps not so committed to a life of crime – or to a personal style and lifestyle in which involvement in crime is a high risk – and are somehow filtered out after release by engaging in more supportive processes, so that they do not re-offend.

There is in effect a form of natural triage, and it is only the ASPDs who continue in a criminal career and hence have a higher representation in the adult prison population. This is a plausible hypothesis, but there is of course no evidence either way. However, with two-thirds of short-term prisoners expected to be reconvicted and to return within two years, and over 90% of under 21s, the need to intercept this cycle of reincarceration is pivotal to any attempt to control the burgeoning prison population.

A final possibility, however, is that the diagnosis and presentation of PD is somewhat malleable. The presentation of personality, including disorderly personality, depends very much on the situation and the relationships with others in which one finds oneself. It is at least plausible that prisoners with an avoidant-dependent or a paranoid personality will decide that if they are to survive in the prison environment and the prisoner community, they will need to look and act a good deal tougher than they are really feeling, and will adopt as a protective measure the ASPD style that they see in the tougher individuals around them.

A somewhat unsophisticated and rushed assessment that takes those presentations at face value may therefore overstate the extent to which it is truly ASPD that we find in the criminal justice system, and to what extent this ASPD-mimicking presentation is better seen as a learned response and even a coping strategy for those that find themselves mired in the system.

I don't mean to suggest that there is a clear distinction here between a genuine PD and a personality that merely disguises and presents itself as ASPD. On the contrary, I want to suggest that the nature of personality, and of PD, is that it is a matter of how people express themselves in their relationships with others, and that some aspects of PD and ASPD are indeed learned behaviours, for everybody with PD – just as indeed personal characteristics are for normal-range personalities.

In other words, it is possible that we may have simply turned the avoidant-dependant type and the paranoid type into ASPD by feeding them through the criminal justice system, without sufficient awareness of the consequences of what we are doing.

At which point, we can turn to the circumstantial and corroborating evidence that we do have to flesh this out into a hypothesis worthy of more systematic research.

For example, a recent initiative in one local authority area (Charnwood Community Safety Partnership, 2010) to explore the roots of antisocial behaviour, leading otherwise to an Anti-Social Behaviour Order (ASBO), discovered that fully one-third of the troublesome youngsters nominated for an ASBO appeared in fact to be on the autistic spectrum. Diversion to family intervention services significantly reduced the rate of ASBOs, and diverted what is otherwise the pathway to a future criminal justice career.

We are, however, familiar with the concept of learned dependence for example. It is not a great stretch to hypothesise a phenomenon of learned defiance. It may be only the fact that responsibility for managing prisoner behaviour lies with the prison service, for antisocial behaviour with the police and housing agencies, and diagnosis with the health service, that has kept these insights apart for so long.

With growing concern at both the human and financial costs of incarceration, and the desperate need to reduce prison overcrowding before any kind of constructive regime to treat the hardened and ASPD core in the prison population, the need to research the characteristics of the new entrants to the criminal justice route becomes acute. Even anecdotal evidence needs a hearing.

Editor's comment:
Staff responses and staff training

One of the issues we are exploring in this book is the extent to which early trauma may later give rise to the chaotic or dysfunctional emotions and reactions that we see, for example, among some people who then slide into homelessness, and/or among those who might get a diagnosis of personality disorder.

One key question is how far we should see the long-term impact of such early trauma in terms of early developmental damage to the brain – following abuse or neglect, for example – interrupting normal development during critical development stages, so resulting in a brain permanently wired for dysfunctional reactions.

Or alternatively, how much might we see the long-term impact more dynamically, in terms of people becoming caught up, enmeshed within social, psychological and emotional patterns that are then very difficult to escape, but which can in principle be interrupted by skilful intervention or even just by good fortune?

For example, is personality disorder – or 'complex trauma' – not so much a fixed, static state, but rather something deeply entrenched in the way people live their lives and their relationships, characterised by frozen vicious circles of repetitive, re-enacted past trauma, now replicated and re-entrenched in self-reinforcing interactions?

One possible way to approach this is by comparison with other areas where comparable issues arise. In relation to learning disability (LD), for example, we can assume that the developmental damage, whatever it may be, has taken place at some very early stage, and at least before birth. Yet the difficulties in living that people with LD have, they have in the present. So it may be instructive to also consider the management of problematic behaviour in LD services.

Chapter 11

The Drama Triangle and other 'unwanted repetitive patterns'

An interview with Susan King

RJ: One of the issues we are exploring is the extent to which early trauma may become, to all intents and purposes, 'hard-wired' into the developing infant brain; or whether it is perhaps more accurate and helpful to think more dynamically and to consider, for example, the seriously dysfunctional behaviour and relationships that we see in people with personality disorders (PDs) as the product of a long sequence of ongoing interactions and mismanagements.

So it would be useful to make some comparison with the management of problematic behaviour in learning disability (LD) services. In LD, as I see it, there is good reason to believe that the underlying damage – if that is the right word – is indeed early, irreversible, and purely physiological. Yet the difficulties in living that people with LD do have, they have in the present, and the problematic interaction issues are ongoing. The contrast may therefore help to highlight the role of other people's responses in helping or hindering recovery.

SK: In LD there will be some underlying irreversible damage. However, people with LD do have personalities, and some people with LD will have PD too. Many others have attachment difficulties, falling short of formally diagnosed or diagnosable PD. LD on its own rarely causes major behavioural difficulties except in severe and profound LD. Indeed the incidence of abuse of children with disabilities is far higher than in children without, so trauma is very often a component of the problems we see in people with learning disabilities.

Much of our work in LD is therefore to help discern what is changeable and what is unchangeable and how best to respond to both. Much of this is done with staff teams and family carers, and more rarely with ward staff, but often with supported living projects or residential homes. At its simplest, the staff and those agencies are being commissioned to manage these things well and so this is where we should focus our efforts on helping them to learn to do things better.

Staff training and support

RJ: Let's look at the question of staff training, because that is certainly one of the areas where the interface between individuals and the agencies is most open to change. Training is the most obvious opportunity to introduce new ideas and to question how things are happening, and certainly training can aim to support or generate reflective practice, which is a huge part of making changes in cultures.

SK: We also have to ask what exactly we think training is. Unfortunately, the call for more training often seems to reduce itself to treating staff as blank slates on which new skills have to be inscribed. We also have to consider how far poor practice, or unreflective services, are really just a matter of the individual staff members' lack of skills, or to what extent it may also be embedded in the culture of the team – what we believe we are here to do; or whether it is equally in the role adopted by the agency. The terms of the contract and the commissioners who fund or purchase these services may also be stuck in narrow patterns of ideas about services and practices that they feel they can't question.

Far too often what you find in 'training' is that staff members are sat down in front of a screen with a series of PowerPoint slides and bullet points and fed information. It is slightly more interactive than reciting the mission statement, but it can be equally disconnected from real life and real learning. Sometimes they are trained in skills such as how to give people choices, or how to engage them in activities, but it is particularly important to realise that staff are not virgin territory and their minds were not blank slates before the trainer walked in the room.

Most people come to care work with some kind of folk psychology, implicit ideas of their own that they have been brought up with and live their lives with. These ideas are generally not elaborated, and rarely put into words, but they affect how staff view the behaviour of those they support and how they feel they should respond. So 'training' may be a misnomer for the process that needs to occur. It needs to be much more of a co-construction of useful models and tools to understand and develop the work, and it needs to take place in a context and a culture of ongoing reflective practice, supported by supervision etc.

For example, one prevailing model we often need to address, expressed in a statement that we hear a lot, is that 'there have to be consequences'. In other words, although it is not generally phrased so starkly, if there is bad behaviour, there must be punishment. This is a strong belief system; all the stronger for being unexamined and unelaborated. I sometimes describe it as poor behaviourism, in that it goes against all the evidence of what works for managing behaviour even within a behaviourist model.

It is rooted as much in a folk morality as in any folk psychology. There is a sense that if people are allowed to 'get away with bad behaviour', a fundamental injustice is done. Of course this is no more thought through philosophically than it is psychologically, but it needs to be addressed often both in terms of 'teaching proper behaviourism', from the psychological angle, and opening up a philosophical or ethical discussion too.

Changing staff's psychological model

RJ: And this doesn't work?

SK: Psychologically, thinking that unwanted behaviour should be managed by consequences simply does not take into account the needs of many people with LD. Their LD may mean they will have difficulty learning from consequences. With some people, their disability is so severe that they really cannot learn new behaviour; in others, it would simply take a very long time. For some, however, their behaviour is driven by its antecedents, its triggers, rather than by consequences, so the behaviour will only be changed if the antecedents are changed. To respond to challenging behaviour with 'consequences' in those situations is naïve, verging on cruel.

Changing the antecedents generally means changing the environment – the physical environment, and/or the social environment. You might ensure the environment is less noisy and overstimulating, or that it is more responsive, or more predictable etc.

Even where people can learn from consequences and their behaviour is consequence driven, we may need to teach staff that to use behaviourism properly, you need to ensure clients get positive consequences for their positive behaviour, especially as the evidence suggests that the lower the person's IQ or developmental age, the more likely it is that they will learn more from positive than negative consequences.

RJ: Could you say a little more about adjusting the environment?

SK: A concept used at times in LD services (and in services for people with brain injury and dementia) is that of the 'prosthetic environment'. A prosthetic environment is one that compensates for the person's impairments, in the same way that a prosthetic arm makes up for a lost arm. For example, making it impossible to look out of the window by drawing the blinds in a classroom to compensate for the attentional difficulties of a pupil with attention deficit hyperactivity disorder is to create a prosthetic environment. To ensure staff plan and manage the budget of people who do not have the cognitive ability to manage their money is to create a prosthetic environment. To give a person with extensive memory deficits electronic memory aids is to create a prosthetic environment.

A prosthetic environment is often distinguished from a therapeutic environment, which would be an environment that is designed to teach new skills, behaviours and ways of being. However, a prosthetic environment may change someone's behaviour by providing them with a sense of security so that they do not need to act out of fear and anxiety. You might argue that both prosthetic and therapeutic environments are enabling.

RJ: It certainly fits well within that broader concept of an enabling environment that we have been aiming to promote. Can we return then to the question of staff training, and reflective practice?

Changing staff's ethical model

SK: You may teach a wider understanding of behaviour management, but this will not address staff's view of justice and how their interaction with clients can demonstrate justice. Getting people to reflect on folk morality isn't easy though. One reason it is so hard is that it is not just at work, it may be how they run their whole lives. If you are saying it might not always be true and right that people have to be punished with consistent consequences, it can mess with staff's heads in so many ways. That person then goes home and they have to think differently about things there too. That's a lot to ask.

If you are looking at the training of staff, and indeed a wider process of supporting their reflective practice, perhaps the most useful thing is to bring into the room the ideas they already have about learning, or justice, or sympathy, or needs. Sometimes just saying, 'This is the world view I was brought up with' is a good place to start. That then allows people to step back and hopefully say, 'OK, this is what I believe, but when I am at work, I may have to consider how different things need to be here'. Rather than simply trying to hammer new ideas on top of old ones, it may be a lot more promising to suggest that we look at how many models of human behaviour we have in the room, and then encourage them to talk to each other. That is a lot more engaging than thinking that people don't have any model in their heads and that they are virgin territory so we can therefore instil a model in them.

Learning to deal with the emotional impact of the work

RJ: We would need to recognise that exposing your own fundamental beliefs to others, even to close colleagues, might feel rather intimidating.

SK: A very important dimension that is often missed is that working with traumatised people is distressing. Yet it is very rare that work is undertaken with staff to address the emotional impact of the work they do, and how to manage that, or the quality of relationships they make with the people they support, and how to enhance that. Indeed, organisationally, the quality of relationship may be poor all the way up the tree. Yet without that, any other training or reflection is of little use.

Generally, in learning disability services in this country most of the training focus is on the skills needed to 'promote independence'. Yet we need to recognise that the emotion of the client affects the staff and that the staff need to manage this, and that there are specific, usually unnamed and implicit rather than explicit and taught, skills that staff use every day to do this.

Professor Carlo Schuengel and his team at the Free University of Amsterdam have an extensive research programme on attachment in learning disability services. Insecure attachment patterns are common in people with learning disabilities, and correlate closely with challenging behaviour. Professor Schuengel and his team have developed a range of programmes to coach staff in the skills of sensitive responsiveness, which they demonstrate can enable the creation of a secure base, and facilitate the learning of new, more adaptive behaviours.

The Drama Triangle: one way of understanding unwanted repetitive roles in care

RJ: Then could we perhaps move onto the notion of the Drama Triangle. It is one example of a straightforward model of the knots people can get into with each other, that can help staff to reflect on their practice, and I believe it was you yourself who first introduced me to this.

SK: Karpman's (1968) Drama Triangle comes from the quite early days of transactional analysis (TA), a way of describing the process also known as psychological games. I find the Drama Triangle useful as a way of simply explaining unhelpful repetitive patterns to staff teams, however it is one of many models of such processes. Others include cognitive analytic therapy's (CAT's) idea of Reciprocal Roles, Karl Tomm's ideas of Pathologising Interpersonal Patterns versus Healing Interpersonal Patterns, or Barnett Pearce's idea (Pearce, 2004) of Unwanted Repetitive Patterns, in which participants feel that they have no choice but to act in a particular way in a particular context.

However, your interest is in the Drama Triangle, so let's explain it here. A 'game' in TA is a series of transactions that is complementary (reciprocal), has an ulterior motive or pay-off, and proceeds towards a predictable outcome. One of the key features of such games is that they are characterised by a switch in roles of players towards the end. The Drama Triangle posits three typical, even habitual positions, which people find themselves taking up in such a game. There is:

- the person who is treated as, or accepts the role of, a victim
- the person who pressures, coerces or persecutes the victim

- the person who rescues ie. intervenes out of an ostensible wish to help the victim.

In the Drama Triangle, the drama plays out as follows.

'[A protagonist] start[s] off in one of the three main roles: rescuer, persecutor, or victim, with the other principal player (the antagonist) in one of the other roles. The Victim is not really as helpless as he feels, the Rescuer is not really helping, and the Persecutor does not really have a valid complaint. Thereafter the two players move around the triangle, thus switching roles.' (Berne, 1975)

The idea is that, for example, the victim turns on the rescuer, or the rescuer switches to persecuting.

Note that the 'game' position of rescuer is distinct from that of a genuine rescuer in an emergency, such as a firefighter or a lifeguard. When played as a drama role, there is something unspoken about the rescuer's attempts, a mixed motive or need to be a rescuer or to have a victim to help. In fact, *'The Karpman Triangle game inhibits real problem-solving ... [and] creates confusion and distress, not solutions'* (Berne, 1975).

The Drama Triangle in care services

The Drama Triangle positions of victim, persecutor and rescuer make particular sense in the care professions, which makes it a useful model to teach to social workers, nurses, doctors, care staff, support workers and so on. The switch – which is so characteristic of games – plays out in the care professions too, for example, when the rescuer is so exhausted by their endlessly fruitless attempts to make things better that they may start to behave in ways that seem resentful and punitive towards the others. So they themselves may perceive themselves as the victim and then behave as persecutor to the others. 'Look how hard I am working with no gratitude,' they might say, 'at least you might appreciate it and not make it too hard – why aren't you getting better?' Alternatively, the victim may harry and denigrate anyone who steps out of the rescuer role, or who does not help them in the right way. The persecutor may then switch to rescuing one of the other parties who has moved to the victim position.

For most of us, a dawning recognition of the Drama Triangle game's dynamic in play will often start with a question such as, 'How on earth did we get into this again?' That is when just knowing the concept of the Drama Triangle can help us then step back and say, 'Hold on – maybe that's what's going on here'.

If any one individual can then step out of the 'inevitable' sequence, it creates some emotional space, perhaps, for the others to do something different too. In TA, and likewise in CAT, the solution is to resist the pull to move into the role that is evoked by the behaviour of the other, and, through reflecting on your own behaviour, to adopt a more neutral, grown-up stance.

The Winners' Triangle

When the Drama Triangle was first proposed, the main conclusion was that workers and others should avoid being pulled into the drama. However, others working in the same TA mode have since suggested more positive responses. In the Winner's Triangle (Choy, 1990), for example, each of the roles of the original Drama Triangle have their equivalent role in a comparable triangular relationship, but the roles of each take a more constructive stance.

Here, the rescuer now adopts the position of caring, and listening; the persecutor aims to be assertive, without blaming; and the victim acknowledges that they are vulnerable and focuses on problem-solving. Whichever player it may be that first attempts to break out of the role in which they have been cast by others – or which they tend themselves to adopt – also aims to use the same reciprocating dynamic to then elicit the matching more positive response from the others in the triangle.

The strategy offered is therefore to take, and seek, the appropriate aspects of each position's emotions, and bring out what is legitimate without over-balancing into blaming others. It is, again, about true assertiveness and self-expression, returned to a more 'mature' or adult position. (In the original terminology of TA, they each say, 'I'm OK, you're OK'.)

Editor's comment: A voice for the victim

For some, 'victim' can be, or can become, almost a state of mind. However, it can also be a strictly formal, technical status – such as for those on the receiving end of crimes. Here, to reduce the long aftermath of trauma, returning some personal control and allowing some self-expression, and the offer of a supporting relationship, seem to be the key to success.

In the criminal justice system, which is focused on apprehension and management of offenders, the role played by the victim can all too easily recede from view and become simply that of a key witness to the crime, or, in the performance management and 'outcomes' of criminal justice, simply a statistic. Some victims of crime have even suggested that their experience of the courts and the criminal justice process can feel almost as brutal and disempowering as the original experience.

To counter this, there have been attempts to offer the victims of all crimes, and especially of serious crimes, the support they may need to come to terms with the trauma of the crime itself. However, counselling and support over their traumatic experience is nevertheless still only one aspect of the needs and rights of the victims of crimes. In more recent years, there have been attempts to give the victims of serious crimes not only support, but a voice in the process of justice itself.

The criminal justice system remains essentially an offender management system, but it is now acknowledged that the victim has rights too, and that the criminal justice system must make sure the victim has an opportunity to put their views forward.

Victim Contact is a service provided by the National Probation Service. Its stated aim is to contact all victims of a serious crime after the court proceedings and the conviction of the offender, to offer the victim information and a channel by which they may have a say in what happens next.

Victim Contact services aim to give them a voice and to make them feel that it has been heard, that their experience is listened to and that it has some weight in the process. The issues that this approach highlights in empowering the victim are explored next, in an edited transcript of a focus group discussion on their work with the staff of the Nottinghamshire Probation Trust's Victim Contact service.

Chapter 12

Empowering the victim in the criminal justice system

Victim Contact, Nottinghamshire Probation Trust

Victim Contact

For every victim of a serious sexual or violent offence (one for which the offender is sentenced to a year or more via the Crown Court) the Victim Contact (VC) service's aim is to offer at least an initial contact – usually a meeting, and usually a home visit – within eight weeks of sentence. That is our target. However the offer is for contact entirely on the victim's own terms. After that initial contact target is met, all other contact is dictated entirely by the needs and wishes of the victims themselves.

That single principle is the key to the development of the VC approach. Contact with and from the team is purely voluntary – and we know that perhaps 50% do engage and take up the offer at that initial stage. Some will decline any contact, others will accept the offer but decline an actual appointment or visit (for whom a phone call and knowing that someone is there may be enough), while others still may ask for contact, but only later, such as nearer the time of release of the perpetrator.

Regardless, all referred victims will stay on the service's books for as long as the sentence lasts. People can therefore change their minds about contact at any time, as long as it is before the sentence has expired. For example, in the case of a very long sentence, after five years the victim might say that they don't need any more contact, and then in another five years they can change their mind. They do not have to be re-referred. Everything is entirely at their own direction.

Before we get involved, there is also the Witness Care Unit. They are part of the Crown Prosecution Service and they take over from the police at the beginning, keeping the victim informed about the process.

A new development

When the VC system started we simply gave information on the legal process; victims did not have any special rights. Now, however, victims can put forward their view via, for example, their victim impact statement to the court at the point of sentencing or via a victim personal statement to the Parole Board when early release on licence, or transfer to a lower security prison, is being considered.

We will listen to their concerns. We can explain to them how the system works and what rights they have, such as their right to request extra licence conditions like non-contact terms or an exclusion zone. We can't and don't promise that they will get their request, but they do have a voice and they can say what the impact on them has been. This is important because now the Parole Board can consider not just the formal legal nature and seriousness of the crime and the prospects of rehabilitation for the offender, but also the impact of the crime.

The reports on the victim's views that we then write can be kept entirely confidential or they can be shared with the offender, and it is the victims who can choose which. Sometimes therefore – for example, for a sexual offence – they may not want the offender to know anything about what their family circumstances are, or what has happened to them, while in other cases they *do* want the offender to know. In some cases that may be a means to saying, '*Now I want to get on with my life*'. Then it becomes their final statement, a part of their own 'closure'.

Furthermore, if they, the victims, do have any anxieties – if for example they don't want the person to approach them – then, as well as helping them put together their victim statement, we can help put things in place to manage those fears. We can help them to write a letter to housing services, to support a move, for example. Giving them information on the process, the points at which they could input, is also part of that. Just taking the time to explain the system can help and you see people visibly perk up. Then it really is the case that knowledge is power.

The nature of the relationship

We are very careful to make it clear that we are not offering counselling – though if that is what they need then we can tell them about services that are available and put them in touch with them, or just talk over with them whether they want to go down that route. We need to have a good knowledge of what support services there are and how busy they are, how long their waiting lists are etc. So although this is not counselling, it can become casework if there are things they need, and you can signpost them towards help. With some people, in the case of very long sentences, you can be involved with someone and be there for them for many years.

While you are not there to be their friend, it is a relationship, and sometimes you might be the only one who actually knows what they went through, or who they can still talk to about it as and when they want to. Then the practicalities of the job are really only the skeleton.

If someone is adamant that they do not need counselling but you can see they are not coping too well then it can become quite worrying. However, if there are problems we are likely to be involved and working closely with the other agencies who are there to help. One year after sentence, if someone is having difficulties, they probably will have other people involved and we are likely to know about it.

VC essentially aims to reassure them that they are not just forgotten and left to their own devices at the point of sentencing, and to ensure that they know that they do have a voice. And again, at all stages, they are in control. We ensure they feel important – that somebody somewhere is taking them into consideration, and they are finally put at the centre of at least some part of the process.

Up until then, apart from the actual crime itself, they have always been obliged to simply play their part in the machinery of justice, which can be a very mechanical process, quite intimidating in its own way. They can't, for example, set court dates to suit themselves; they can't affect the legal process. Every other experience they have had has involved them going to other people on other people's terms. With our service it is the other way round.

That is why it is so important that we can visit people in their own home where they can feel comfortable and are in their element. You can have a cup of tea in your own cup, without having to ask someone else's permission and use someone else's cups. Little things like that you might hardly notice, but they make all the difference. It may be the first time the criminal justice system has ever gone out and wrapped itself around you.

It is important that VC is, and remains, an actual part of the criminal justice system because it is the system itself owning the need to make a place for the victim in it. It is not a separate service, cut off from the serious, proper business of offender management. It is an integral part of it.

Of course, it helps in practice too that we are insiders – we know how the system works, or at least how it should. There is an issue that the culture of the criminal justice system needs to be changed here, and it is not always easy. If we are part of trying to make a place for the victim's views, we sometimes have to be quite assertive with our colleagues about what the victim has a right to know and when they should be told. As we are insiders we know the ropes, and if something has not happened when it should, we can push maybe more than an outside agency could, certainly more than a counselling service could do. Furthermore, because we have a good understanding of the whole system we can sometimes take shortcuts and can get through where an outside agency might not be so well placed to.

The public face of the criminal justice system

Sometimes we do have to deal with some quite inappropriate behaviour – the kind of language or attitudes that with anyone else, in any other situation, you would not tolerate, for example from someone who is contacting us because something about a case has not gone the way they wanted. People can get very frustrated and scream at you on the phone, such as when we have to give them bad news, for instance when an unexpected early release date is announced.

Then it is like being a punch bag. Often it is not us they are angry at, but the whole system, but you have to take it. That is the point of giving them a voice.

Then there is the diplomacy. We sometimes have to tackle attitudes from other people in probation and there can be some quite stressful relationships or communications with other workers in the system. It can be hard when we know a victim's rights but the other worker just does not get it. It is amazing how many offender managers we have to have quite forceful discussions with to get them to see things from our perspective – even just reminding them of the rules and regulations they should be following.

It is like we are bringing a different way of working into a system that does not want to change. Obviously people's own values come into this, and some people just do not believe that the victim's views should have any weight in the criminal justice system. However, we are the ambassadors for the victim, and that is about changing the culture.

Coping with the stress

To help us manage we get external supervision support with a trained counsellor. It is not counselling, but it is for our own support – the VC and the offender managers who deal with the most serious violent and sexual offenders. As you can imagine, they have to deal with some pretty fraught situations too.

We also have a way of getting support from each other – it is like a code for '*I need some help*'. Sometimes one of us will just ask a question out loud and the others who are there will ask whether it is a question for anybody or 'a question for the room'. If it is the latter, however busy we are, all the chairs swivel round and we chip in with any advice or thoughts we might have. The burden is therefore spread around the team, and everyone is very supportive.

The physical space of the office helps that a lot. The set-up we have now works because we have a space where all the liaison officers are in the same room, and we are separate from the more open plan area where the offender managers sit. There may be confidential things we have to discuss, which we would not want to share – and nor would the victims. In a completely open plan office or a thoroughfare we could not share and support each other in the same way. You would not get that closeness.

Previously we were on the ground floor of our HQ building, which was a thoroughfare and the manager was in a separate side room. It just did not work. When the whole large county service was splitting into local units on local authority boundaries, the original plan was to have one worker for each area, with the Offender Management team for each area. We argued, based on our experience, that it was important that we were together, that this gives us a strength, and so we stayed as a unit. That has been an interesting bit of learning for us – what a difference it made.

If we were split into locality teams we would be completely lost because there would be nobody you could bounce ideas off, nobody that would understand it from your point of view, because their role is very different. In fact, we had a colleague who used to come over or who would phone us up to get some support, among people they knew would understand.

We have since shared that with colleagues in other areas, where their service has chosen instead to split people up, and we can also pass this up to management here and to the national office.

Editor's comment:
Working within the culture of an organisation

The experience of victims of crime is a timely reminder that trauma can occur in people's lives at any time and that working with trauma is not just concerned with early trauma. The example of the Victim Contact service again touches on the role of social institutions in managing and containing powerful emotions. It indicates the enormous efforts that it may take to introduce a new element in the overall culture of an organisation, even in some small and relatively marginal area.

The example of Victim Contact also shows the necessity of placing the vulnerable and traumatised individual at the heart of a service, and as far as possible in control of their own part in it – even if sometimes that can only be achieved by creating a small new area at the margins of the rest of the service, where a different culture can grow.

Our next two examples indicate the importance of recognising and working, where possible, *with* the culture of the organisation or social group, and developing and supporting natural resilience.

Chapter 13

An occupational hazard:

managing traumatic incidents in the fire and rescue service

Viv Brunsden and Laura Lawrence

'Team support needs to promote rather than interfere with the group's natural recovery and coping ... The support mechanism should provide a safety net for the minority of individuals who need more than the support and help that peer groups offer.' (Lawrence & Barber, 2004)

Emergency services personnel, such as firefighters, police and paramedics, are routinely exposed to traumatic experiences as part of their daily working lives, thus putting them at risk of developing symptoms of post-traumatic stress or even post-traumatic stress disorder (PTSD). This has led to a growing recognition within these services that there is a need for occupational health teams to put in place well thought through programmes of trauma support, to buffer this exposure and alleviate any negative effects.

Indeed, employers have a legal, as well as moral, duty of care to their employees when their work involves them engaging in situations that place them at risk. This creates a complex therapeutic situation, as employees may on occasion need to be referred for interventions on a mandatory rather than voluntary basis.

The approach most commonly linked with the emergency services is Critical Incident Stress Debriefing (CISD). This is an approach that involves the entire group of exposed personnel in a facilitated discussion, providing them with the opportunity to work through their experiences and feelings related to a specific traumatic event. Initially seen as a positive step forward in managing stress and trauma, CISD has somewhat fallen out of favour in UK emergency services, following a widely publicised report, a Cochrane Review (Rose *et al,* 2002), that raised doubts about its efficacy.

However, it now seems that this negative conclusion may be based on a misreading of the evidence. For example, the wider literature on CISD has also to take account of crucial variables that can have important effects on its efficacy, such as:

- how soon after the event the CISD debriefing took place
- where it occurred (specifically in terms of whether it was delivered at, or away from, the event)
- whether it was voluntary or mandated
- who were the population being helped.

The last matters because, as Jacobs *et al* (2004) note, while CISD can be ineffective for accident survivors, it can be highly beneficial for emergency service personnel.

Another crucial variable that the literature review did not consider was whether the CISD was peer-led or professional-led. Yet our research shows that emergency service personnel can be extremely resistant to external professionals. The internal culture of the services leads to a strong occupational identity; one which believes that those who have not experienced the sights, sounds, smells that emergency services personnel themselves have, can never understand their experiences.

Perhaps, however, the most important variable that the negative literature on CISD has failed to take account of is that such interventions always operate in a context. Like most therapeutic or other interventions, CISD is rarely applied in and by itself, but instead is usually just a single strand of an overarching Critical Incident Stress Management programme (CISM). The original Cochrane review (Rose *et al*, 2002) considered only single-session CISD interventions, whereas in practice most CISD programmes utilise multiple sessions.

Like CISD itself, CISM as a wider context for interventions can take a variety of forms. In the UK fire and rescue services (FRS), one method, which has become known as 'the Tyne and Wear approach', is gaining a reputation for positive practice in this area (Lawrence & Barber, 2004). The basic premise of this approach is the recognition that, following traumatic exposure, both individual and collective coping mechanisms will naturally and organically come into play. Any homogenous group has an implicit set of understandings by which it operates. These will usually include a level of self-help, by which emotional defence mechanisms are activated to protect the integrity of the group when a threat is perceived.

Formal interventions take time to organise regardless of how well an organisation is prepared, and natural coping processes will always have had an opportunity to begin. Attempts to intervene should therefore aim to start with these, and avoid anything that might disrupt or undermine these natural rhythms and processes that form a crucial part of the resilience of emergency service personnel.

For operational personnel within the FRS, the most crucial 'natural' support network is 'the watch'. This is the group of people who work together as an operational team. They share the same experiences and act as one another's first line of debriefing and diffusion. Remotely involved people, such as control room staff, are also exposed to potentially traumatising experience while taking calls. In terms of exposure, their involvement will be different to that of the site responders but they have potentially endured a highly stressful event, and need to be offered the same support.

However, this natural small group support may not be enough and people may wish to discuss things outside of this group. The Tyne and Wear approach acknowledges that need, and therefore offers a tiered support mechanism that begins with encouraging this natural peer support, but then allows individuals to self-refer to the in-house Trauma Support Team (TST), for a trauma support session (a TSS). Members of the TST are volunteers who continue to perform their roles as emergency services personnel while undertaking this additional TST role.

The TST offers support in their own right but also act as a form of triage, that is, they can refer people on for professional therapeutic interventions where need be. They undergo a rigorous selection process to ensure that they have the personal qualities needed for the role, and are themselves psychologically robust enough to take it on. This is needed because there is a strong awareness of the possibility of secondary traumatic stress and the need to also care for the carers, and in this way, the health of TST members, as well as those they support, is safeguarded. It also means that ordinary FRS staff can have confidence that the TST volunteers are to be trusted.

The TST undergo an intensive in-house training course to equip them with the basic skills and knowledge to conduct TSSs. During this course they are continually assessed before being offered a place on the TST. This is followed by at least 12 months' experience observing the team as they facilitate TSSs, shifting over time to facilitate the sessions themselves under the supervision of experienced team members. During this period they have to keep a learning journal recording any influences upon, and continual critical self-reflection of, their own practice. Each new member of the team also has a competent and experienced member of the team who acts as their mentor.

The second part of the training is delivered by The North East Trauma Centre. This deepens team members' practical skills as well as increasing their levels of theoretical knowledge. The training borrows from the cognitive behavioural therapy (CBT) model and incorporates such elements as Socratic questioning, feedback mechanisms and more in-depth knowledge of conditions such as PTSD, depression and panic.

Following a further six to 12 months' practice with the team, the final part of the course is then undertaken with Northumbria University. This final stage allows team members to investigate the relationship between, and integration of, academic theory and workplace practice. This external training also allows them to gain a Professional Practice Award and is available at both undergraduate and postgraduate levels.

The training programme is therefore a unique and valuable tripartite development between Tyne and Wear Fire and Rescue Service (TWFRS), The North East Trauma Centre and Northumbria University. Taking this approach has ensured not only that the scheme exactly fits the needs of TWFRS, but that it adds to the experience and qualifications of TWFRS personnel, adding wider value to TWFRS as a whole. Perhaps most importantly though, it endorses the importance of the services of the TST, confirming the status of their work. It demonstrates that team members' actions are appropriate and professional, while still sitting entirely within the service itself.

This is important because the FRS can be extremely resistant to 'outsiders', particularly in terms of support for psychological distress. One form that takes is the aforementioned belief that someone who has not seen, heard or smelled the things that they have could never understand how they are feeling. Using peers as TST members breaks down this barrier, and training them to professional standards ensures the support is as appropriate and professional as any outside agency could provide.

In this context, it should also be noted that there is still some mandatory referral within the approach. If an incident results in two or more fatalities, then referral to the TST is compulsory. However, this is no longer resisted by personnel because of the cultural shift within TWFRS where the notion of trauma carrying any stigma has effectively been removed.

The issue of stigma relating to traumatic reactions is an important one. Current research (Sanderson & Brunsden, 2011) into the armed services, which share many occupational risks and organisational structures with the FRS, suggests that while personnel may say that stigma around trauma has been removed, in practice this may not be the case. Although fully accepting that people who have faced terrible experiences can be traumatised by these, and would therefore need help, when armed forces personnel were asked if they would ever need or access such support they gave a very firm 'No!'. (See Chapter 14 for a further discussion of trauma in the context of the armed forces.)

It appeared that their 'acceptance' of traumatised reactions applied only to others; for themselves, they still demonstrated the stigma attached to post-traumatic stress, characterising such reactions as a sign of unacceptable weakness. This internal stigma, that arises from the individual's self-image has apparently proved immune to the changes brought in by the armed services. By contrast, the Tyne and Wear approach appears to have removed not only the wider organisational stigma but also this internal stigma, allowing personnel to take control of their own health and to freely engage with support systems.

One possible reason for the difference between the reactions seen in personnel from the armed services and at TWFRS may relate to concepts of 'organisational self'; an identity exclusively based around one's sense of belonging to an organisation or occupation. Both sets of personnel have been found to have extremely strong organisational selves in terms of a strong identification with their specific occupational role. However, there is some evidence that firefighters' organisational selves go beyond this and have a shared collective identity, seeing themselves as a 'universal firefighter' (Hill & Brunsden, 2009). This identification of the self, as standing collectively with all other selves who are firefighters, means that any stigma applying to a single firefighter would also apply to all firefighters. This means that, if stigma is removed from others, it must necessarily also be removed from the self.

The sort of trauma encountered during work, the experiences faced by servicemen, paramedics, firefighters etc, is necessarily different in key respects from other forms of trauma. Traumatising experience *per se* is rare, unusual or unexpected, passive and individual. However, those in response roles, such as firefighters, are likely to have cumulative traumatic experiences, with these experiences being expected, even planned for, and actively engaged in rather than passively received. These are likely to be highly significant factors for resilience.

However, they can also become barriers to seeking help when viewed as an occupational inevitability. An individual may feel they should be able to cope because it is 'merely' part of their job. The Tyne and Wear approach gives permission to those who need additional support. The need to access additional support is not seen as an occupational failure or as any threat to the identity of the organisational self. Instead this need emerges from the collective organisational self, as that necessarily carries a responsibility for mutual and individual care. Support thus becomes about good health practices and centres on well-being rather than reflecting any form of stigmatised illness.

The introduction of this approach at TWFRS, focused on empowerment, peer support and health, has been supported by careful efforts to develop the internal culture of the organisation. The organisation as a whole, as well as the individuals within it, are encouraged to accept that traumatic exposure is inevitable and that experiencing stress as a result is perfectly normal rather than a sign of weakness. An educative programme has been running alongside the enhanced trauma support service. This has been supported and co-delivered by the Fire Brigades Union.

TWFRS is convinced that since the introduction of this approach sickness through traumatic exposure has reduced. More importantly perhaps, the views of those who have self-referred are entirely positive. There is a definite change in the culture seen within TWFRS. In other fire and rescue services, the still 'macho' culture can make acknowledgement of psychological distress very difficult, which forms a serious barrier to help seeking. In TWFRS this barrier has disappeared and people talk freely about stress and willingly self-refer.

Elsewhere it has been argued that services working with vulnerable people, such as some homeless people with complex needs, may need to develop as psychologically informed environments (see Johnson and Haigh, 2010), and this approach is now endorsed and recommended (CLG/NIMHE, 2010) for resettlement services, refuges and similar services. The TWFRS experience now suggests that the introduction of psychologically minded support, especially where able to work with and within the existing culture of an organisation, can introduce elements of a psychologically informed approach into other environments where stress and trauma need managing effectively.

In recognition of the pressures that firefighters face, The Firefighters Charity developed a telephone support line. This was intended to provide easily accessible support not only for the firefighters themselves, but also for others connected with the FRS, such as their families. These families may be dealing with the difficult reality of living with a stressed family member, and they need help too, just as much as the firefighters themselves.

This evidence of the need for support for family members led the Highlands and Islands Fire and Rescue Service to commission the Nottingham Trent psychology team to look at this issue of support for families (Hill & Brunsden, 2007). The mechanisms in place for them were multifaceted, bearing all the traditional aspects of social support. However, a key finding emerged that families wanted initiatives such as newsletters and discussion forums specifically for the families, ones that could be set up *by* and *for* the families.

Editor's comment: The price of vigilance

Another area where traumatising experience 'comes with the territory' is in the armed forces. Soldiers on active duty must not only face the stress of being under fire, they may also face the hidden threats of mines and booby traps – improvised explosive devices. If constant vigilance is the price of freedom, it is the frontline service man or woman that must pay much of that price.

Perhaps most difficult of all, they must also learn to put aside any qualms about shooting back, and shooting to kill. Considerable efforts now go in to managing this emotional journey – though for some, the journey back may be the hardest part.

There is currently considerable public concern for the fate of ex-servicemen who leave the armed forces and return to civilian life.

Chapter 14
The traumas of war

Combat Stress

Mark Smith and Robin Johnson

In 2011, on the back of a report requested by the Prime Minister, David Cameron, into what support was available for veterans of the armed forces, the Department of Health commissioned a confidential telephone helpline for veterans.

The services charity Combat Stress, from their knowledge of this group, advised that the helpline service might need to operate with a style rather different to that of other helplines, with their careful neutrality and a concern for professional distance. For example, to engage with this new client base and ensure that the callers are at their ease, it has been agreed that helpline workers may adopt an informal and more engaging approach that is more in tune with the culture of the armed forces and the language that is used. The Combat Stress 24-hour Helpline is now in action, provided by the mental health charity Rethink Mental Illness, in conjunction with Combat Stress.

Within days of opening for business in the early summer of 2011, the helpline began receiving calls from serving personnel in active combat zones. It was immediately agreed that this was a need that could not be denied. The service also readily takes calls from family members worried about their loved ones and listens to their concerns.

The helpline service is still new and rapidly developing, and making every effort to make itself available to currently serving and former service personnel. For example, the service is now expanding to engage potential helpline users initially via email and text – all still fully confidential. This reflects both the need to be available over long distances and to distant time zones, and the opportunity to work with new media, which reflects the age group and character of the high-tech culture in which the service is engaged.

The hotline is already breaking new ground in developing innovative approaches, to deliver valuable support and positive, de-stigmatising 'messages' about mental health to areas where there is most work to be done – the armed forces and service families. In addition, they are already in discussions with a university regarding the prospects for research, in looking at the wider lessons that might be learnt from developing this new style and methods.

'You look out for your mates'

In a conflict zone, service men learn to rely first and foremost on each other. They look out for each other, mind each other's backs. When servicemen are de-mobbed, they carry with them the experiences of war, and for many, traumatising flashbacks and other vivid and disturbing memories. Now, however, they must face these memories without the key feature that gave them the resilience to manage the challenges of combat – their mates. Their greatest strength is the thing they must now do without.

When in the services, their life is organised for them – their accommodation, their meals, their daily routine. It is all too easy for the daily living skills needed for 'civvy street' to wane from disuse, and on discharge, having to suddenly fend for themselves can be a shock in itself.

One of the practice examples used in the 'complex trauma' homelessness guidance was that of Home Base, a planned treatment environment in North London for homeless ex-service personnel with psychological difficulties, run by Community Housing and Therapy (CHT) Trust. Here the approach is described in more detail, incorporating direct quotations from service users.

Base camp

John Gale

Homeless people with a service history are more likely to be assessed as having mental health problems than the general homeless population – 39% compared with 26% (Johnsen *et al*, 2008). Many of those who are referred to Home Base suffer from complex trauma, depression or anxiety, or post-traumatic stress disorder (PTSD), and will have become homeless, partly as a result of the psychological problems they experience. A number have a diagnosed personality disorder. These problems are frequently exacerbated by alcohol or drug abuse, unemployment and inadequate life skills. Nearly all will have a very limited support network, lack self-esteem, feel worthless and find it hard to form relationships.

CHT has an approach to the therapeutic community that stresses the central importance of belonging to a community as the essence of the therapy. The full CHT programme consists of four distinct but overlapping and interrelated treatment interventions, with individual counselling and group work. But the programme is designed as a whole, as a psychologically informed environment, in which each element complements and supports the others.

First, the programme is fundamentally designed as a community in which all aspects of the social and physical environment play a part in the treatment. Rather than focusing on individual psychopathology, the approach focuses on the interpersonal and social context of psychological disorders and well-being. The group functions at the interface between the social and the individual. The value of the group, which acts as a container into which projections can be made, also encourages sharing responsibility and participating in decision-making. This enables service users to support one another in the process of recovery (Hinshelwood, 1987).

Second, group psychotherapy sessions focus on the relationship between symptoms, behaviours and unconscious factors (Gale *et al,* 2008). The aim is to enable service users to understand their experiences, particularly those traumatic experiences from their military service, and to link these with earlier experiences of trauma, especially those in early childhood. This relies on the development of a secure attachment with other members of the community.

Third, cognitive behavioural therapy (CBT) is used to influence dysfunctional emotions, behaviours and cognitions through a goal-oriented, systematic procedure. CBT interventions aim to restore a more optimistic outlook about the future and those that develop communication skills are particularly effective with complex trauma and PTSD sufferers who tend to avoid discussing the traumatic event.

Fourth, the programme places a strong emphasis on training for work. This aspect of the programme is run in partnership with Training for Life, Transitional Spaces and other organisations that assess employment skills and deficits, and arrange courses and placements for homeless people and former members of the armed services.

In the Home Base programme, the community structure encourages participants to share responsibility and participate in communal decision-making. This enables ex-servicemen to support one another in the process of recovery. It values and builds upon members' experiences of solidarity with comrades under fire, but uses this to develop the skills to live outside the military.

The following excerpt is from a group discussion with half a dozen tough and battle-hardened men, all of whom live in their own one-person flats, either in or clustered around a housing complex. These men were clearly not overly comfortable with the idea that what they received, or needed, was in any way a form of therapy. Nevertheless, what they have to say speaks for itself, and illustrates the importance of recognising the fine line between group therapy and peer support.

'When you're in the services, you're taken care of and it's like your little bubble. As soon as that disappears, you feel daunted and isolated. There's just nothing there, and your bubble's gone. But here, it gives you that little sense of belonging that you're missing, maybe.'

'There's things you can talk to one person about that you wouldn't feel comfortable sharing in the group. But the main thing about the group is that you get different stages of people who are left. When I first came, a year ago, the group was about eight people, and there was some who'd been here two years, all the way through to me, who's just arrived. I was like the new boy going to school.'

'...and you're, like, "oh lord, what's happening?". And just to talk to you normally, and bring you in, and let you know how it will work, was the good thing. An individual chat with your specialist, your therapist, whatever, can't do that. But as a group, as we are now, then, when you get together, if you get someone coming in, and you can bring them under your wing slightly. And it actually gives them something to go, "Okay. I feel a bit better now. I'm not so ... you know..."'

'I know if I ever had a major problem I could pop up here and speak to someone, or phone, and we've got each other's phone numbers and that. There is always each other. Even though we have our own lives.'

Editor's comment:
Rebuilding self-esteem

The examples of Combat Stress and Home Base provide further perspectives on the issue of trauma as an occupational hazard, and the importance of working, where possible, with and within the cultures of frontline service personnel, rather than simply offering standard therapy or counselling. The Home Base example in particular suggests that there is a very fine line between therapeutic work and other equally enabling relationship building. When working with a service culture that takes pride in resilience, this can be a very fine line indeed.

We will return to the role of peer support and enabling communities in two later examples, in EXACT's work on recovery communities for individuals with problems of substance abuse, and Rex Haigh's 'one-stop shop' personality disorder development in Slough.

For the moment, we should also note that the post-war therapeutic community movement itself has its roots in the resettlement and rehabilitation services devised by the army for traumatised and institutionalised British soldiers during and immediately after the Second World War. Some of this history is told in Section three.

Rebuilding self-esteem is also a key theme in the next example, which returns us to the issue of homelessness and the sometimes chaotic lives and histories of people who find themselves homeless. It would be wrong to think that homelessness services simply provide shelter and a bed. The Department for Communities and Local Government/National Mental Health Development Unit guidance (2010) gave many examples of deeply engaged and constructive work being done by dedicated services working with some of the most excluded people in our society.

Here we can go deeper into this area than the many brief vignettes given as exemplars in the guidance itself. Here, Peter Cockersell of St Mungo's describes the service users he has worked with and the issues that they have lived through. Peter's psychodynamic framework is informed by contemporary understandings of human difficulties arising from the neuroscience of trauma.

However, in blending this together with the concept of personal recovery, Peter's paper echoes that of Fraser and Webb's work in the Romanian orphanage (see Chapter 5), in challenging the idea that early trauma becomes fixed for life, and demonstrates that there is no point at which we can say that damage is permanent.

Chapter 15

Homelessness, complex trauma and recovery

Peter Cockersell

Who we are and where we come from obviously informs our perspectives. I will therefore begin by introducing myself. I had a fairly troubled youth and was asked to leave a few schools before finally choosing to leave at 15. I spent a few nights on the streets, took a lot of drugs and alcohol, engaged in antisocial behaviour, and had some happy but ultimately damaged relationships.

I am now a psychoanalytic psychotherapist and have worked clinically with homeless people and people with complex trauma for over 10 years, in the NHS, specialist surgeries and day centres. I have worked with homeless people in various social care roles for almost 20 years, and I am an operational director of one of the larger voluntary agencies that works with homeless people. I could regard my own life, therefore, as an example of the capacity for recovery that I mean to describe.

The homeless people I have worked with over the years come from almost every imaginable background, and each has their own unique history and experience. They are not homogenous, but they do have some things in common. There are, for example, very high levels of emotional and psychological disorders, diagnoses of mental illness and drug and/or alcohol dependency (Maguire *et al*, 2010; Cockersell, 2011). There is a disproportionate frequency of complex trauma among homeless people and rough sleepers, or what could equally be described as chronic or compound trauma, with incidents going back to infancy or earlier, and then recurring through long periods of the person's life.

However, homeless people and rough sleepers also have the fact of their homelessness in common. This too, in many people's experience, is not a singular episode or event, but a chronic series of experiences. They will often have long histories of unsettled and changing accommodation, with little positive experience of 'home'. One 50-year-old man has had an astonishing 88 moves in the last 40 years. The number itself is astonishing, and so is the fact that he has kept count, which seems indicative of the impact it has had on him. 88 moves is not just unstable accommodation – homelessness on this scale is also a state of mind that makes settling anywhere very difficult.

In a very useful discussion, Scanlon and Adlam (2006) conceptualised the 'unhoused mind' and drew out some relationships between chronic trauma and long-term or acute homelessness (eg. rough sleeping) among some people with borderline personality disorder. Myself, I think 'unhomed' mind might be a more exact epithet. Some people have very negative experiences of 'home', and so it is a dangerous place, to be avoided. Some have such an unsettled concept of home that it is always somewhere transient and prone to be lost.

Although all histories of chronic trauma, homelessness and recovery are deeply individual and particular, there are recurrent themes that illustrate actual processes and that can help our understanding both of why people remain homeless for so long – how they become 'entrenched', in the jargon of homelessness agencies – and also why and how they recover.

This chapter will look at some of these histories of complex trauma, homelessness and recovery. The histories come from five different individuals either currently or recently using homelessness services. They were among a group of people who volunteered to participate in a study of the experience of homelessness (Cockersell, 2010). They have all very generously agreed that I could share their stories and my analysis of them. Their names and other details are changed.

I will identify some recurrent themes in their stories, and use them first to illustrate the links between chronic trauma, mental health, substance use problems, and homelessness, and second to illuminate the mechanisms and interventions that positively impact on and support recovery.

Complex trauma and homelessness

'*No man is an Island, entire of itself; every man is a piece of the Continent, a part of the main.*' So wrote the poet John Donne (1624), and modern neurobiological and attachment research strongly supports this perspective. We are significantly shaped, particularly in terms of our brain physiology and its expression through our 'personality' and our 'mind', by our early (perinatal and infantile) developmental experiences (Schore, 1994; Siegel, 2011) and through the impact of our primary relationships.

Indeed, we are not only shaped by our own experiences, but by the experiences of those close to us. There is, for example, evidence of a link between behavioural disorders in adults and prenatal bereavement in their mothers (Liotti, 2007).

One client I worked with grew up while his father was in prison for attempting to murder his mother when she was pregnant with him, a difficult legacy to live with, especially as his mother found it hard to express love for him and used to frequently tell him how like his father he was. He refused to work, refused resettlement, refused support, yet remained in a hostel with 24-hour support and dependent on benefits: he was determined not to become an adult man like his father.

There is now a wealth of literature on the links between the experience of trauma and emotional and psychological disorders (eg. Solomon & Siegel, 2003; van der Kolk *et al,* 2009), and between the experience of trauma and what health and social care agencies coyly call 'challenging behaviours' (Batmanghelidjh, 2006). The disproportionate levels of emotional and psychological disorders, mental illnesses, substance dependency and attempted suicide among the homeless population are also established.

- Around 60–70% of the homeless population meet the criteria for personality or post-traumatic stress disorders (Fazel *et al,* 2008; Maguire *et al,* 2010), compared to five to 13% for the general population (Department of Health, 2009b).
- 30–35% have diagnoses of severe and enduring mental illnesses (Timms & Fry, 1989; CHAIN, 2009; St Mungo's, 2010), compared to around one per cent of the non-homeless population (Department of Health, 2009b).
- 61% are substance dependent (St Mungo's, 2011), compared to around 5.5% of the non-homeless population.
- 42% had attempted suicide in a survey of 1000 homeless people (Bonner *et al,* 2008), compared to a European average of 1.3% (Bernal *et al,* 2007).

What then may have led to such levels of difficulty? A study of homeless people in Sydney found 90% of men and 100% of women (Buhrich *et al*, 2000) had experienced trauma, including over 50% of women and 10% of men having been raped. The numbers of men who have been raped is, for obvious reasons, likely to be under-reported. 74% of clients of a homeless psychotherapy service reported either childhood abuse and/or neglect, with high levels of early traumatic loss of a parent or caregiver. Furthermore, 24% reported sexual abuse (St Mungo's, 2011) and 11% of all St Mungo's clients have been in care (St Mungo's, 2010).

There has not been, as far as I know, a published systematic study of the experience of early and chronic trauma among homeless people. Despite the lack of systematic studies, the prevalence of emotional and psychological disorders, of psychiatric illnesses, and of substance dependency, alongside what data there is and the personal accounts by homeless people themselves, all provide persuasive evidence for the strong link between complex trauma and homelessness.

So how does it happen?

Five case studies

Let's look at the stories told by our five volunteers. I present them with a caveat: inevitably, in the space available I cannot do justice to the richness of meaning of their personal histories, nor more than hint at the feeling that was expressed in their telling. These are the bare outlines of these people's stories.

A's story

A's parents put him into temporary care when he was four, and then never took him back again. His father was a sailor and his mother said she could not manage him alone. He lived in a succession of care and foster homes before joining the army for a couple of years as soon as he was old enough. After leaving the army he did casual work and sometimes stayed in lodgings.

His father died in an accident abroad, and when A was 22 he was told by the Salvation Army that his mother had also died. He has visited her grave once. He had lost touch with other family members by then. He stayed in various cities before ending up in London, where he stayed sometimes in homelessness hostels or shelters, often being moved on, sometimes leaving because he did not like the noise or drugs. On and off, he slept on the streets, because, as he put it, *'sometimes it's better on the street'*.

In the 1980s he got married, having met his future wife in a day centre, and lived with her for 17 years in her flat. One morning he woke to find her dead in the bed beside him. This prompted a nervous breakdown and he was hospitalised. The council repossessed the flat, which was in her name. When he left hospital he went back to living between the streets, hostels and shelters for another 10 years.

He still gets depressed sometimes, *'but not every day'*. He is confident he will move into sheltered accommodation shortly, but he will continue to visit the project he is in now because *'they've been so good, you can't forget people like that'*. He has become attached to them.

B's story

B lived with his parents together in the same place for the first 10 years of his life; they then moved to another area. *'I really felt it'*, he said, and described being the *'odd one out'* after his move. His parents separated two years later and he lived to and fro between them. He also sometimes lived with an aunt, but he had to keep the relationship secret because his mother didn't like her. His mother neglected him, often not even feeding him so that *'feeling uncomfortable inside'* seemed normal. She *'was always bearing a grudge'*, he says, *'a bit of a sadist, doing things to hurt you'*.

He worked a lot, mainly in driving jobs, and moved frequently (B is the client who has been in 88 places in the last 40 years). He had a big relationship, his 'true love', which lasted a few years. But then his father and his aunt died and his 'true love' left – all in the space of a year. He had a relationship with another woman, Joan, that became abusive, and lasted *'four years too f***ing long'*. He moved abroad and severed contact with everyone he had known. Despite a bit of casual work, he became homeless because, he said, *'of despair'*.

He was living in a bus shelter when he started hearing voices and seeing visions of Joan. He was voluntarily hospitalised abroad, and then returned to England and to rough sleeping. After a while he was hospitalised here too, put on anti-psychotic medication, and given a diagnosis of schizophrenia (the onset of which he attributes to the abusive relationship with Joan). He then moved into a hostel. He did write to his mother, who is still alive, but her reply contained *'as many sadistic references as you could get in'*, and so he tore it up.

He still has occasional nightmares, and sometimes hears voices, but he likes where he is living (supported housing, just around the corner from the first place he moved to at the age of 10), and feels *'more settled'* than he has before: *'I go to bed in peace,'* he says, *'and I wake up in peace'*.

C's story

C lived with his parents until he grew up. He went to work and had a good steady job with a big company. He got married and had two children. He was close to his family, and especially to his father and daughters. He liked a social drink with his mates in the pub or while watching football, but he never caused any trouble.

Then, however, his wife ended their relationship after 19 years, for reasons he would not talk about. C went to live in another town, got another job, and found a new girlfriend. Upon the death of his father soon after, C left his new relationship, moved back to the city of his birth and went to stay with his mother. He continued to like a social drink. Although he had a seizure that frightened him, he did not really associate it with alcohol.

After a year, though, his mother made him leave, and said she didn't want him living there. He went to live with one of his daughters. She asked him to leave after a couple of months, after which he went to live in a drinkers' hostel, which, as he put it, *'wasn't the best scenario, drinkwise'*. Health problems, however, and a couple of bad falls, insistent but caring pressure from his daughter who still visited him, and the birth of a grandchild, led him to the realisation that he *'could stop drinking and solve so many problems at once'*.

With help, he did. He is now dry, working, living in a flat, and in another relationship.

D's story

D's parents separated when she was little after her mother had an affair with another man who her father tried to murder. He also hit D and beat up her mother. He was arrested and she and her mother went to a refuge. After they were resettled, her mother formed a new relationship with a man who used to beat her, and raped her for a period of several years. When she ran away to her father's he beat her up too. Eventually she ran away to a cousin, who looked after her.

She did well at school, got a good job and married a wealthy businessman with whom she was very happy, most of the time, for five years. Sometimes he was violent though, and he sometimes forced her to have sex when she did not want to. Then his business got into trouble, and one day she came back from work to find that he had disappeared with everything in the house, including clearing out their bank accounts. She attempted suicide and very nearly died.

She sees the experience as the beginning of a change. There *'are no limits once you've died'*, she says, *'you can create yourself as who you want to be'* because there is *'no fear'*. After being discharged from hospital, she spent three years homeless, living mainly in hostels. She is now in a supported house, waiting to move into a flat, and she has just got a professional qualification and is looking forward to going back to work.

She still sees her parents sometimes. Her father has developed Alzheimer's, which she told him would let him understand some of the mental anguish she had been through. Her mother lives alone, and D visits her sometimes. The cousin who looked after her died recently, but D saw her the night before she passed away and she told D that she had always counted her as one of her own children.

E's story

E was born in Africa. His country was torn by war and when he was around the age of nine the police took his father away; he never saw him again. He does not know what happened to his mother either and he cannot even picture her face any more. He, his two brothers and his sister escaped to England where they were granted refugee status.

They went to live with an aunt, but she said she could not cope and brought in social services who split the family up. E was very upset about this, describing it as heartbreaking. He was rehoused with his sister and he very much liked the foster mother they were placed with. However, after two years, social services decided to move him again because the foster mother 'wasn't a cultural match'. This time he was separated from his sister as well.

He got into the *'wrong circle of friends'*, began to drink and take drugs, and *'almost drunk [himself] to death'*. His sister paid for him to go back to their own country where he found work and met someone who had known his father. He wanted to come back to England, however, and returned when he had raised enough money. He came back to live with his sister: *'Things were alright for a while'*, he says, but his sister *'had changed'*. After he began to feel troubled, and then to hear voices and feel paranoid, he went to his GP who referred him to the Community Mental Health Team and they gave him a diagnosis of schizophrenia. His sister asked him to leave.

He is now on medication and social services arranged for him to move into a supported housing project for people with mental health problems. His psychiatrist and Community Psychiatric Nurse are, he says, *'brilliant people'*, because they talked about real feelings. He now wants to *'move on from the past'*, which is like a *'blur'*. He is sorry for his older brothers who *'witnessed a lot'*. One is in and out of prison now, while the other has a gambling problem.

E is now waiting to get his own flat, which he hopes will be a fresh start. *'You have to have some belief in yourself ... to survive'*, he says, *'and though life's knocked me down, you have to choose not to give up'*.

Links between trauma and homelessness

In each of these cases, traumatic experiences preceded homelessness, and in each case there was more than one traumatic experience, often within a short space of time. Furthermore, in each case the impact seemed to be more than the individual could deal with: C became homeless out of despair. A, B and C all moved away from the places they had always lived. D tried to kill herself, B and E got drunk, and A, C and E developed mental health problems that triggered long-term psychiatric interventions.

The traumatic experiences all involved their nearest and dearest. A was abandoned by both parents before he was five, then had a series of care and foster homes, with every move adding further loss. B was left by his wife of 19 years who took their children, and then his father died. C was neglected by his 'sadistic' mother, lost his friends and social network, his parents split up and he moved from place to place and person to person. D's parents separated when she was little; she was hit by her father and raped by her stepfather, and then abandoned by her loved but abusive husband. E lost both parents by the age of nine, then his country, then his brothers, then his sister, and the foster mother he loved, all before he was 16.

This is a staggering amount of loss in the lives of just five people, with much of it experienced before they were even adult.

It is reasonable to speculate that, given their personal histories, the experiences of compounded attachment stress that our five clients experienced were sufficiently extreme to trigger some very basic emotional defences. The degree of loss was not survivable – it was experienced as overwhelming, it felt as though it could not be processed or lived with – and so each of these clients in their way refused to accept it. It is as if their conscious, self-aware selves could not at the time assimilate the experience. Some got drunk, some ran away, some developed psychoses, some tried to destroy themselves. All became 'homeless'.

The old expression 'home is where your heart is' contains a truth: home is where you feel loved and where you are with those you love. Without love, a room, flat or house is only accommodation, not a home. Some homeless people have never experienced a stable, secure home. One client who I asked what home meant replied, *'my mother's blood spraying across the wall'*. He stayed homeless all the time I knew him, and would never settle anywhere.

These five clients became homeless because they lost those they cared for. First they lost their mental and relational sense of home, and then became physically homeless in the sense of being without secure accommodation. In a way, their homelessness was a communication, as if they were telling everyone what had happened – they had lost the spaces and relationships within which they had felt, or should have been able to feel, safe and loved. They were too traumatised by their losses to recognise the root of their distress.

From this analysis, providing accommodation is not the answer to the 'problem of homelessness' because homelessness is often, indeed usually, not a problem of housing. One outreach worker said to me that for many of his clients *'being on the streets isn't the problem – it's part of the solution'*. The 'problem' is one of severely damaged and damaging relationships, and a damaged capacity to relate.

In some cases, providing accommodation, especially the 'self-contained unit' prioritised by many housing commissioners, regulators and legislators, is actually likely to reinforce the person's sense of loss, isolation and fear. Indeed the most common reasons given by resettled homeless people who go on to abandon their flats are loneliness and isolation. The appropriate response to homelessness, then, is to foster improved relationships and/or capacity for relating. Experience supports this analysis: where we have tried this approach, using individual psychotherapy to help people clarify some of their relationship issues (often a missed process of mourning), the results, in terms of people moving on, are very positive (Cockersell, 2011).

Similarly, specific positive relationships (notably group relationships) are cited as key components of initiating and enabling their recovery by homeless clients who have successfully moved on (Groundswell, 2010). Of our five volunteer cases, A and B cited hostel staff as of crucial importance, C cited his daughter and his new partner, D and E cited their psychiatrists, D her cousin and E his community psychiatric nurse and keyworker. They all spontaneously talked of individual relationships that were crucial to their recovery, and they all also talked about the importance of groups of activities.

Trauma, homelessness and recovery

It is no coincidence then that there is also strong evidence that positive relationships are critical to recovery from trauma (Solomon and Siegel, 2003). There is now very good evidence that trauma shapes people's minds and relationships (Schore, 1994). However, the great plasticity of the brain and the dynamic nature of the mind continue to make change achievable (Siegel, 2011), as demonstrated by the many amazing recovery journeys of homeless people. Positive relationships, and the positive interactions that accompany them, directly stimulate the neuronal growth that facilitates personal development (Siegel, 2011) and enables stability, maturity and the ability to move on (Goleman, 1998).

From this perspective, providing support for recovery from homelessness for many homeless clients is in fact about providing a physical and relational environment in which it is possible to recover from attachment stresses created by complex (or rather compound) trauma, through positive relationships. Just as a child needs a relationship with a primary caregiver to be able to process the 'bad objects' that otherwise get split off and become destructive internal or external fantasies, so the traumatised homeless person needs the positive relationships that provide the safe emotional environment in which they can process their losses.

Once the unacceptable or overwhelming trauma can be processed, they will be free to successfully move on and to return home, or to find a new home. Until this processing is done, home cannot be found because home is in a mental space that cannot be reached. This manifests itself in the frequency of homeless clients 'sabotaging their resettlement' by some behaviour or other.

Developing positive relationships and managing relationships positively should therefore become the 'bread and butter' of homelessness staff, rather than being an add-on or something that specialist staff might do (and even then only when there is time). It is no exaggeration to say that relationships are at the core of recovery, and of effective provision for homeless people. There are many ways to create an environment and working practices that foster positive relationships, such as incorporating mindfulness, emotional intelligence, co-production, reflective practice and many other concepts and techniques.

An approach that attempts to co-ordinate many of these is the psychologically informed environment (PIE). Very useful guidance has been published by the Department for Communities and Local Government (CLG) (Keats *et al*, 2012), and there is supporting guidance from the CLG/National Mental Health Development Unit (2010) and the Royal College of Psychiatrists (Johnson & Haigh, 2011a) material on 'enabling environments'. I have described elsewhere (Cockersell, 2010; 2011) the process followed by the agency I work for when adopting this approach. Recovery research also contains much about ways of developing positive relationships and of deconstructing some of the power dynamics that can easily bedevil institutional and professional relationships (Shepherd *et al*, 2008).

In summary, in many or most cases homelessness is not a housing issue, it is a consequence of complex, chronic and compound trauma that simply becomes too much to bear: home ceases to be a helpful or safe concept. Chronic trauma impacts on brain development and that in turn impacts on behaviours and social relations. These are compounded and reinforced by chronically unsettled and/or actively hostile experiences of home. However, recovery is achieved through a series of positive social processes that enable a mental redevelopment – a reframing of brain and mind – that in turn enables the creation of another narrative and an alternative future.

Relationship building is therefore at least as critical a response to homelessness, and to the recovery from homelessness, as housing itself. Positive relationships heal trauma, and so enable us to find or re-find our 'homes'.

Editor's comment:
Manageable chunks of time

The previous article illustrates the compounding of traumas in the lives of Peter's clients, and the emotional vulnerability that means that early difficulties can so easily reopen. However, it also shows graphically the power of individuals to engage in deep change and the importance of the relationship, as another kind of 'scaffolding'.

Psychotherapeutic counselling is a very effective way to engage. Nevertheless, there are other ways that may seem initially more superficial, yet can be equally creative and thoughtful. One such approach is based on the idea that people with chaotic lifestyles may find it easier to manage tasks with short time horizons, and if we can find ways to make possible these immediate rewards, then the sense of achievement derived can provide a platform for re-engagement on which to build.

'[For users, being] in recovery from problematic drug use is very hard to imagine, both in terms of how to undertake that journey and in terms of what a future life could look like. In fact, neurobiological research suggests that damage done to the frontal lobes by chronic drug use affects users' capacity for a 'memory of the future', the ability to see or imagine future options. Among young people in particular, there is a substantial time-preference operating: the long-term, uncertain potential costs of drug use are discounted against the immediate benefits of taking drugs, which works in tandem with people's natural optimism bias about their own life course. Only when people start to enter employment, for example, do perceptions about the future become longer.' (Daddow & Broome, 2010, pp 137–138)

As in the youth work approach at St Basils, working with disorganised people's limited time horizons could certainly be seen as psychologically informed, and working with their aspirations fits with the overall direction of humanistic psychology, which intentionally appeals to people's creativity and strengths just as much as it works with their problems.

In the following example, the Potter Street 'TimeBank', we can see once again the importance of working with short time horizons, and supporting efforts in personal change that build upon self-directed growth. However, the example of Potter Street also serves to show that – as with playwork – not all therapy needs to look like therapy, and it can have many faces.

Chapter 16

Banking on time:

Potter Street TimeBank

Graham Gardiner

In our local homelessness service we have developed several initiatives that engage with clients in many ways beyond simply finding them a place to stay.

Of course, many immediate tasks involve resolving the immediate accommodation needs of the clients, but the launch of a new hostel in Worksop brought new challenges. Here we had a group of fairly chaotic heroin users, many of whom had been given the label of personality disorder (PD), most of whom had never stayed in a hostel, and many of whom were pilloried by the local community.

One of the solutions we came up with was to develop a TimeBank – a concept based on what was originally an American idea (Edgar Cahn's 'Time Dollar' (Cahn, 2004)) – and firmly in line with the Asset-Based Community Development model that formed the basis of much of my own work.

The basic idea is that people would use their time and talents in return for time credits, broken down into 15-minute chunks, which could then be used in exchange for various services, just like money. The standard unit of time in TimeBanks is usually one full hour, but we reduced this to 15 minutes because our client group were particularly chaotic, and getting them to focus for any extended length of time was setting them up for failure. In terms of redesigning any service, you really have to get a handle on who your customers are.

We decided to run a range of activities for people to earn time credits, because we realised we needed to prime the pump of talents; it wasn't something that came naturally or that people found easy to do.

They got credits for cleaning around the house (double credits for the toilets at the top of the stairs), sewing patches on jeans or cooking the Sunday meal, for example. In fact, anything we could think of we rewarded with time. The most popular was getting up to £5 off their personal rent charge. Every week we used to play football against one of the local drug agencies – everyone who played got credits. It was great as a way to break down the barriers between users and the workers. If we won, they got double, and I used to pay people to turn up as supporters.

It was really interesting to see the change in the way the neighbours saw our clients. We wanted to use the TimeBank to connect with the local community, bringing a new range of challenges and opportunities. We did deals with a local community centre to accept TimeCredits for their three-course lunch. The community centre in turn then used their TimeCredits to get some of our clients to help wash up or clean. A local charity shop entered into the spirit and offered clothes in return for TimeCredits.

There was one local vicar, however, who didn't get it. When delivering the parcels from harvest festival, we insisted he take TimeCredits in return. After initially refusing, he eventually relented but said he had no need of them. Even a strident polemic about the Church engaging with the people I housed failed to win him over – until two months later that is, when he desperately needed volunteers to set his church hall out for a function!

We then realised that we could use the TimeBank even further, to help motivate certain clients who were most stuck. For example, we had one young man who always said he wanted to go to college, but he was demotivated and disorganised, and so we paid in time credits for him to go, just for one month. By the end of that month he was in the habit of doing exactly what he had actually wanted to do but had been unable to motivate himself to do it.

We had another tenant, a particularly chaotic and traumatised female heroin user whose room was always covered in needles. It was very unsafe and by rights we should have chucked her out. But instead we offered her a deal: we paid her in time to get to the needle exchange and when she realised she could use that to pay off her rent, and keep the cash, she started turning up every week handing in her needles and getting fresh ones. This made her, and us, feel a great deal safer.

Some people were critical, saying we were just giving people an easy life or keeping them dependent. We were acutely aware of that. However, we were actually trying to give people new habits. I am a great believer that you just need to break the cycles, and sometimes you need to be very focused to do that, and be very tailored to the individual. This is a complex issue in terms of equality, and often we might have one client saying, *'It's unfair – she got this'*, and so we would respond, *'Ok, well, what would work for you?'*

If you work with a person-centred approach you simply can't be consistent. You need to be honest and transparent, and say: if you have a need, we will work something out with you. It is fair, because we will be inconsistent with everybody, and that is a kind of equality, after all.

We then started getting people to do things for each other. For example, we had a client called Jane who was good at filling in forms, a task that otherwise the staff would have to do, and so we thought why not pay her in time? This soon caught on and people began to ask, *'What can I do?'* and we might respond, for example, *'Well, there's a garden...'*. It didn't really matter what, the point was to remind people that they have assets.

We had one guy who cooked breakfast but he made far too much, and he came to the office and asked what he should do. So we told him: sell it. Work out how long you spent on shopping and cooking; divide that by half – because you are eating half of it – and offer it to someone who hasn't eaten. After that it all took off. You can't plan for situations like that, but we created a culture where it was possible.

We had great fun with it; it was playful. People will engage with you if they can see that you are passionate and having fun, otherwise they will think you are just another institution and it won't work. We had one member of staff who was particularly inventive and so we made her the 'Time Broker'. We created time in the rotas for her to do that work; just a couple of hours a week. There was a free bit of kit that you can download and so we were even able to give out bank statements!

Were we a psychologically informed environment? Not formally, because all this really comes from understanding what was going on for the people. My understanding was that I had a bunch of people who didn't feel valued, who didn't feel they were worth anything and that they had nothing to offer. In fact, this was exactly what the local public were constantly telling them – and sometimes to their face, quite forcefully. I don't know what model of psychology that would be, but it seems to me that we did have to challenge that negative image. We needed to say that people are valuable, they have assets, they *are* assets, and we need to help them find that in themselves.

The day we realised that our TimeBank was really making a difference to the lives of our clients was the day one woman, a 23-year-old with a six-year heroin habit, paid off £5 in rent, had lunch, bought some clothes and then had her hair done for the first time in years – all using TimeCredits. She came back to the hostel with a big smile and looking great. Even better was that she told the hairdresser that she had done some hairdressing courses when she was younger and that she'd like to volunteer for him. And he paid her, of course, in TimeCredits, which he earned doing other TimeBank participants' hair. Here were people furthest from community life contributing, being recognised as assets and helping themselves in the meantime. It really worked.

The beauty of it is that it is cost-effective. In the organisation I worked for there was a pot of money for service-user involvement initiatives. We had to bid for it, and we won £5,000 to develop this. After two months I gave the whole lot back because we simply didn't need it. What we were doing was paying for itself. I think that if you are creative, you can do this stuff.

Editor's comment:
Substance abuse, relapse, and 'outer strength'

In the examples above we have looked primarily at what people can do for themselves, and how services of various kinds can help them do so – to find their way out of the self-replicating spirals of trauma. The model that Potter Street drew upon for inspiration is called 'Asset-Based Community Development', and we will see the same idea taken forward in the example that follows.

First, however, we must also look at what people do that does not work, both individuals and services. Foremost among these are the issues that arise when individuals attempt to ameliorate relationship stresses, frustrations and still more tangled emotions by self-medicating with drugs or alcohol.

This is not to suggest that all substance abuse arises out of deep-seated or early emotional trauma – as we have seen, traumatising experiences may come at any point in an individuals' life. Yet it seems likely that substance abuse – and especially increasing reliance on substances for relief – disorders any personality.

In work with substance abuse, until recently treatment services have tended to reside within hospitals, or for more extended work, in specialist therapeutic communities. There remains a tendency in statutory health and social care to focus primarily on such intensive, intentional treatment-model services for those who need, and who recognise the need for, intensive support.

However, what of those who have passed through treatment and detox, and now face the challenges of living with sobriety? What are the fundamental anxieties in drug and alcohol recovery, as distinct from the short-term containment of an inpatient detox?

Here, the psychological and psycho-social issues are somewhat different from those in treatment services. For those who have tried many times to stop their habit, the greatest fear is of slipping back and of finding all the other myriad daily troubles of life just too much without the solace of a drink, a smoke or a fix.

For those all too aware of the powerful lure of oblivion, one of the greatest enemies is denial – the human capacity for self-delusion when faced with temptation. When a fragile resolve and lonely ego-strength have failed to be enough time and again, it is no surprise that many self-help programmes in substance abuse turn to a power outside of the self (James, 1902; Alcoholics Anonymous, 2007).

However, this 'something outside the self' need not be a mystical 'higher power'; it can also be other people. We know the power of group membership to help people stick with a difficult decision (Lewin, 1948). Here, the issue is how to rebuild one's life, how to remake a new identity and a new social circle – for street drinkers, the street and the bus shelter are often the only community they have – and, in particular, how to live in the permanent shadow of the risk of relapse.

Not surprisingly, here too housing and community networks have been, for some, a part of the solution. 'Dry' houses for recovering alcoholics and 'clean' houses for ex-users have proved an effective response to the real emotional issues of keeping the faith, and sticking to the decision to live differently. These are existentialist communities, where every day the individual must retake the decision to stay clean, or stay dry, and the fellowship of others is an invaluable resource.

Such houses provide further examples of the benefits of developing communities in order to provide peer support, with peer-responsibility and peer-confrontation not replacing but complementing solitary struggle. This is, after all, the essential core from which the therapeutic community movement once grew, and it should not be forgotten that the concept of recovery originated in self-help treatment for self-identified alcoholics.

Still, this is a tiny percentage of the total population of those with problematic substance abuse. The majority either do not need or would not accept such intensive living arrangements. With hazardous alcohol use becoming a major public health concern, we need perhaps to think of new ways of creating enabling environments for the majority of people with such problems who continue living in their own homes.

What follows is an example of a radical attempt to go beyond traditional and limited approaches whereby ex-users contribute to the development of services for those with substance abuse issues. This is an extract from a presentation by Brian Morgan, service user project co-ordinator with West Sussex Drug and Alcohol Action Team at the opening of Studio House, Nottingham.

Here, Brian describes the creation in West Sussex of EXACT – from 'Ex', meaning 'experts by experience', and 'act', meaning, 'to do something about it'.

Chapter 17
Building recovery communities

Brian Morgan

In West Sussex, we at the Drug and Alcohol Action Team (DAAT) wanted more input from service users to inform their commissioning – that is, we wanted people to tell us what they need, what works well, and what does not. We could have simply set up some tokenistic service user group consultations and left it at that, but from what I had learnt in my time there, I knew that that is not the best way of doing things.

Instead, from the start, we set up the service user groups as independent community organisations in their own right, and that is what EXACT is – a network of groups. Because the EXACT groups are independent they can do what they want themselves, and because they are community groups they can fundraise for whatever they want to do, and quite a lot is not to do with drugs and alcohol at all.

The network we created now does two things: service user involvement, as we were originally tasked to do, and building recovery communities.

Recovery community is what I've been asked to talk about, because that is what, in reality, we are doing. This is an approach based on the principle that it is the people who need and receive services who are the experts. This is how we put this idea into practice in West Sussex.

When we first started, we went into partnership with the Royal Society of Arts (RSA) who were interested in seeing how to redesign services from more of a service user point of view. (An account of this whole development is available on the RSA website.) The origins of EXACT were in what was originally called the User Centred Drug Services Project.

West Sussex is a large county with a varied geographical landscape. It has an extensive coastline, large and small urban centres and miles of rural land. As well as having areas of affluence, the county has areas of extreme deprivation including Local Neighbourhood Improvement Areas that receive supplementary development support. Parts of the county have some of the highest rates of alcohol related hospital admissions in the southeast region.

With such a population dispersed in pockets, we first set up a number of local groups. EXACT has six local hubs covering seven county districts:

- Adur and Worthing (one EXACT group covering two district council areas)
- Arun
- Chichester
- Crawley
- Horsham
- mid-Sussex.

Each group is part of the West Sussex Forum, which is the central point for the network of peer led groups. This offers a huge amount of first-hand knowledge and experience and meets once a month to work together to develop the groups' capabilities and strengthen the network.

Eventually we had over 200 service users in West Sussex involved in the design of the service, and sure enough these service users said they wanted services to be more peer-led and more flexible. They wanted things to be open outside working hours and they suggested quite systematic changes to make things easier to access.

None of this was completely new. However, one thing that was new was that the idea that the whole focus needed to be on recovery, and not just on treatment; about life outside of services. In services, and then in service user involvement, more often than not people will sit around and talk about substance use. In contrast, in recovery, more often than not people talk about things that are not related to substances.

The recovery concept was therefore coming in to the whole system – and there was a creative cultural shift away from traditional services. (Incidentally, the service user project co-ordinator job description from 2009 does not once use the word recovery, so the world really is changing quite a lot, quite quickly.)

As the RSA (Daddow & Broome, 2010) themselves put it:

'Our project was conceived as a way to build and test personalised services with recipients, couched in a recovery framework. What soon became apparent was that our emphasis needed to be reversed. Personalised services generally exist within a traditional framework of service provision. But recovery is ... grounded in the community and ... is a transition that can occur without professional input, and where professional input is involved, the extent of its role is far from clear.'

In the end, what we designed was what we now call a Whole Person Recovery System. That is, we set up a recovery-centred system, rather than a treatment service and a total rethink of how it all fits together was also needed. Quite often people get well without ever going into treatment, just by being in their community with support from family and friends. We came to the realisation that recovery and community is where treatment sits, not the other way round. Treatment is not the solution, wellness is. For that, you need others.

We need to start building recovery communities, and building them from the ground up. Of course, recovery communities existed before treatment, in Alcoholics Anonymous, Narcotics Anonymous, therapeutic communities and the like, and many are based in peer support fellowships of one kind of another. The 'new' communities should include them, and a lot more besides.

It can be any group of people who have being in recovery in common. They are out there already, although sometimes informally, and it is all about bringing them out, bringing them together and building them up. EXACT is an umbrella group to support the creation of local groups and link them.

You start with getting like-minded souls together and then commence what is called in the trade Asset-Based Community Development – conveniently shortened to ABCD. ABCD is a different and powerful approach to developing communities and the people within them. It starts from the idea that all communities have the potential to be rich – they all have assets and resources which, uncovered and mobilised, have the power to transform.

This 'glass half full' attitude challenges the embedded deficit approach favoured by many public agencies, and it encourages people to take an active and proud role in turning their lives and communities around. It provides a space where people can build their confidence and capacity to bring about positive, lasting and sustainable change.

How does it do all that? Supporting and encouraging people to uncover their own potential and those often-hidden resources that are already available to them is transformational. Individual and collective confidence grows, and communities can go on to identify real areas of unmet need. Active and empowered, with their own resources and assets working for them, they are in a stronger position to access additional external resources and to put them to most effective and sustainable use.

First, you start with yourself – what have you got? You look inside yourself. What are the good parts, what are your strengths and assets that you can put to use?

Then, what have you got within the group as a whole? What have you got between you?

Then the rest of the community – what can you get to use? There might be a library, a minibus, sports clubs, volunteering of all sorts, local events and festivals etc. We have found that a 'recovery' cafe is particularly popular with recovery communities.

You start with yourself, but it can't stop there. You want to be making a network – grow it up and grow it out. Once we start, recovery is contagious – you catch it from each other. The person who passes you recovery is the same person who passed you a £10 bag. But instead of the contagion of addiction, we can start building the contagion of recovery.

Contagious recovery rests on the premise that if individuals socialise with people who are 'healthy' they are more likely to become and remain healthy themselves. EXACT has a very important role to play in generating pathways from cultures of addiction to cultures of recovery.

We are doing it with EXACT in West Sussex, but now, with the UK Recovery Foundation (UKRF), we are trying to build these networks across the whole of the southeast of England. The UKRF envisions a world where the power, hope, healing and potential of recovery is thoroughly understood and embraced within communities, society and support agencies. A world where people, families and communities affected by alcohol and other drugs will be enabled to find their own solutions, their own empowerment. A world where people will be supported to access the support they need to achieve recovery, health, wellness and emancipation.

These communities will form the constituencies that will do three things:

1. Ensure treatment remains to be seen as a sound investment.
2. Scrutinise the performance of commissioned services.
3. Become a support network in their own right that can 'hold' people in recovery once there.

Most importantly, the development of recovery communities – through EXACT in West Sussex for instance – is of benefit to all involved in drug and alcohol issues in local areas. It will build the constituency that will be needed when power is devolved to local decision makers. For far too long we have all taken the funding of treatment and services for granted (commissioners, providers and even service user groups). These communities will provide the evidence that it should continue into the future.

Editor's comment:
The community dimension

No one wishes to suggest that all people with severe drug or alcohol problems are suffering from a fully developed personality disorder (PD). On the contrary, for those long-standing problems of substance abuse, it is particularly hard to tell where the personality issues end and the addiction issues start. Nevertheless, there is a striking similarity in the lifestyles and problems described by many of the users of the EXACT service with those histories found among others who become homeless, or among those who do acquire a PD diagnosis.

There is also a striking similarity between the account that Brian gives of the progress of EXACT and the direction being taken – or perhaps found – in some of the new PD services that have been spinning off from the original 11 Department of Health pilot services set up after 2004. In the next chapter, Rex Haigh describes the fast-moving pace of development of the PD service in Slough.

Chapter 18

A one-stop community

Rex Haigh

There's something happening in Slough at the moment that is very relevant, and which shows how the health service can still be creative and open. This is the story of how we have made it so over the last two years, although I think that the last two years is nothing compared to what the next two years will bring.

I had been away from Berkshire for a few years, helping to set up therapeutic communities (TCs) in other parts of the country as part of the Department of Health pilots, when I was asked if I would return to my own employer and set up a fairly small scale, minimally staffed service, as a local 'spoke' for a service with its main hub in Reading.

Reading is home to the Winterbourne Therapeutic Community, which was the original template for non-residential TCs in the UK, and has since been copied and modified in various other locations. It was set up in the 1970s when it was located at the county asylum (Fair Mile, in Wallingford), but converted into a modern personality disorder (PD) service by Jane Knowles, Jean Rees and myself when we moved into suburban Reading in the mid 1990s.

However, the approach we took to developing this new local 'mini-service' in Slough was different and quite exciting. I had decided to begin by simply gathering a group of people who might benefit from the kind of programme I was familiar with and that we had been setting up elsewhere over the past few years.

I had an office to use in a health service building alongside the psychological therapies team, who were there delivering properly evidenced PD therapies (mostly dialectical behaviour therapy) in a competent and caring but rather conventional way. (After all, if they are to be properly evidenced therapies they have to be rather conventional. It comes with the territory of having a standardised and manualised procedure that you then apply.)

We started off meeting for half a day once a month, running it almost like a focus group rather than any kind of therapeutic programme, asking service users what services they had or hadn't had. We provided lunch to create that sense of breaking bread together, making it all very sociable, and otherwise did the usual TC things of group discussion, group ownership of the issues that came up and dealing with the hurly-burly of different voices and views.

We then moved into a phase where there were enough of us to meet weekly. We still had the same intention to make this the planning and preparatory phase for setting up a three-day programme. Eventually there were about 12 of us meeting every week, including one rather bewildered senior occupational therapist and myself, with two 'experts by experience' on loan from the Oxford-based Thames Valley Initiative. The meetings took place in a 'Friends meeting house' – a Quaker meeting hall – which is quite a nice link when you think of how in the UK, way back in the Napoleonic era, it was the Quakers who had started off humane psychiatry at the York Retreat.

We were planning something that was not the old-fashioned and rigid TC model, with highly structured programmes and a focus exclusively on therapy. What was of central importance was establishing a certain culture, a 'quality of relationships' if you like, and the mechanical details of when, where and how often were secondary issues. Although in fact there are no residential TCs in the NHS now, and very few five-day programmes, the one in Slough is one whole day, and two other groups during the week. It is really very minimal and people do things themselves at other times, outside the meeting programme. It is really their time – although we insist it is cohesively held together, and that the individuals are all well supported within the network of containing relationships between them.

The group was immediately surprised by the fact that they were being asked about things, rather than being told what was good for them. They were sat down, given a cup of tea and asked their opinions – being treated as human beings, rather than being expected to sit outside in a hospital corridor or in a waiting room, and called in half an hour late for their appointment and so on. This, remember, was officially still the preparatory phase, but most of the emotional work is done in getting to the point where you are ready to do the work. I would tell them that if they could just come each week, just turn up, that is all they have to do. They are all now so bored with me saying that!

It was about a year before we started the full programme, the traditional non-residential TC: a community meeting at the beginning and at the end of the day, and in between playing games, going for walks and so on. It took off in a way that could sometimes be really hairy – people went right into heavy duty therapy straightway, and we sometimes had to help pull people back from jumping in at the deep end before they had learned to swim.

When we have visitors, the service users just love telling people how different this is from most mental health services, and they say so in a way that is so eloquent, it knocks me for six every time I hear it. It's not me doing it, or saying this, it's them – they are doing it for each other, and with each other, with a depth and method that very few statutory services would understand – or perhaps tolerate.

When we moved to the hospital (when renting external space became an expense the NHS would no longer cover) the only place available for the regular programme was a doctors' seminar room in which we 'squatted'. Our temporary home was where we did nearly all our therapy for the best part of a year. In fact, we kept getting kicked out, having to vacate it for various 'more important' reasons. You might well imagine the sort of emotional response this generated in the members of the therapy group.

We are now about two years into the project and we have a fully functioning three-day programme and have gathered together over 10 staff (and more than 10 who have had secondments or voluntary and temporary contracts with us). I am the only person actually paid to deliver the service. The others are all on loan from other services or are volunteers, ex-service users or psychologists wanting some experience before they go off to train. Sometimes they might only be able to commit to being there one day a week, or even just one half day, but they all have proper agreed roles, are all called social therapists, and they are assigned to particular groups. We are a virtual team – we communicate through posting notes for each other on a secure web forum after the meetings. We therefore have a wide range of staff without a clinical team – a seriously minimal service.

However, that is not what is so different here. I have set up communities like this in the past – this is in fact the seventh TC I have set up. This one was different though. As well as the groups and the usual hurly-burly, we had a policy right from the start that we would always accept professional visitors. We let it be known to all sorts of people out there in the community locally – and some came from beyond, to see what we are up to. Almost every visitor is impressed by what they see, and these visitors have included quite a lot of people from local communities that deal with a lot of people with PD, such as housing social services, child protection and probation (we have people from housing, but not from homelessness – at least not yet).

Several months ago two people came from the local council's chaotic families team who were so interested that they wanted to stay for six-month placements in order to learn about group work. They have gone on to do group analytic training in London, and we are now well advanced in drawing up detailed plans for partnership working as a 'one-stop shop' for people diagnosable with PD in Slough.

This all fits very well with the Knowledge and Understanding Framework (KUF) training, with teams of services users and clinicians delivering the courses. The people who have been through the programmes that have been going much longer than us (Reading, Oxford, Aylesbury, Milton Keynes and others) are now KUF trainers, and they are helping to make Community Mental Health Teams, acute inpatient wards and various other settings into more therapeutic environments. So now we have set up different social enterprises (as community interest companies) to deliver training and services in this field, hopefully – ultimately – in partnership with the NHS trust, using local authority and health funding, as well as housing, education, justice and others.

It is increasingly becoming this 'one-stop shop' for PD in all sectors in Slough. It is very circumscribed, just this local area covering a small urban, deprived and ethnically diverse population, but it is for anybody with those sorts of problems. And we are hoping to expand and to keep growing, not just as a standard TC, but with a range of activities, therapy groups, community events, and social experiences – all preferably in a 'greencare' setting (Sempik *et al*, 2010) – somewhere with horticulture, some looking after animals, arts and crafts, and other 'low-tech' activities that put people in real contact with nature.

I want to explain and promote how this model crosses barriers and can bring together different agencies under a common therapeutic philosophy. It's not really about the specific techniques that people bring, it's the common ground of building it from the ground up with services users, across agencies, valuing the relationship.

There's one last twist. We have seen a site we're interested in but I don't know if we will manage to get it. However, almost jokingly, I had said to the medical director of the trust that the one thing that would help us keep people out of hospital – those who in a crisis have nowhere else to go – would be something like the Haven PD pilot service in Colchester. There they have a nice big building with about 150 people on the books coming and going by day and a number of crisis beds (the Haven has six beds) for service users. We are expecting a decision any time now about whether or not they will put this in the development programme.

Editor's comment:
Housing, home, community

The widening of focus, from the individual to the community at large, is occurring not solely in the recovery communities that Brian Morgan describes in Chapter 17, but is a theme that is now being picked up with enthusiasm throughout the healthcare community. In his 2004 report, *The NSF Five Years On*, Louis Appleby, then UK national director for mental health, argued that *'we need to broaden our focus from specialist mental health services to the mental health needs of the community as a whole'* (Department of Health, 2004).

At a moment in time when depression has taken over from back pain as the most common disability identified in Incapacity Benefit claims, we, as a society, need to begin to address the 'common mental health problems' of anxiety and depression. However, the 'burden of ill-health' from depression is not the only area of concern for community mental health. We may now need to look again at how best to address issues such as substance abuse, trauma, personality and stress disorders.

This does not need to mean that our already over-burdened secondary care services must throw open their doors and become all things to all people. Nor does it mean a huge expansion of mental health services, which would surely create impossible expectations, and would also inevitably provoke accusations about the 'medicalisation' of ordinary human distress.

Instead, if we are serious about developing a social model of disability and a focus on social inclusion, we need to look outside the specialist mental health services to see what the rest of the community has been doing to respond to these issues. This new vista may reveal a very different future direction for community mental health care.

Chapter 19
Trauma in later life

Robin Johnson[1]

We have defined psychological and emotional trauma as the overwhelming impact of challenges the individual cannot process. However, any full consideration of the interplay of trauma and social context for the most vulnerable needs to include the risks for the old as well as for the young and the socially marginal.

However late in life, traumatic experiences at moments of greater vulnerability can have a most devastating effect on the individual's life, and the ageing brain is, in its way, as vulnerable to trauma as the developing brain of the infant or the maturing brain of the adolescent. Then, equally relevant to these questions are examples of enforced life transitions such as those met by the isolated elderly in changing communities, and especially of the devastating impact of care home closures for those with dementia. Both are, at different levels on the trauma scale, about the needs of those without the resources to cope with change over which they have no control.

As life expectancy increases, and the population ages, we may need to consider the ordinary stresses impacting upon the mental health of older people – not just of those with dementia, but those many older persons for whom the principal common mental health problems are anxiety and depression. Worries over loved ones; worries over failing health; fear of increasing dependency, and a wish not to 'be a burden'; dwindling finances and rising fuel bills; loneliness and isolation as family members move away and communities change; and especially loss – of their role, of loved ones, of shared references and common history. All too often, these are the day-to-day experiences of older persons.

However, if these might be seen as mental health issues, then we can see the extent to which the development of such services as warden-aided accommodation units is actually a very well tuned and effective response. While taking care – particularly in 'extra-care housing' – of a person's physical needs, they primarily address their social and emotional needs by providing safety and security, peace of mind, company and companionship, and opportunities for caring about and for each other.

---

1 Part of this article first appeared in *Mental Health Today* December 2007 – January 2008 pp27–29.

The growth of extra-care housing over the past 10–20 years has demonstrated (Darton *et al*, 2011) how popular and effective this kind of integrated care can be in maintaining individuals with all the dignity of independent living, and also the very real benefits of living with congenial company. In the private sector, gated 'retirement communities' have also been one of the fastest growing sectors of the housing market.

As the health benefits of social capital are being increasingly recognised, so the healthcare gain from shared living housing options becomes clearer. In both gated and sheltered accommodation we find a community dimension that promotes peer support, befriending, and even mentoring.

In the words of Mary Bryce (2007), director of care services at the Housing 21 housing association: *'This is not just housing-related support. These are housing-based solutions to community care needs. What we are providing here is a real community, not just a building with services in it.'* These are practical, purposive responses, services allowing the older person to remain in control of their own lives as far and as long as possible, attempting to ensure that ageing and increasing physical frailty is not stressful and debilitating.

Transition trauma

There have been highly influential studies clearly demonstrating that allowing residents in care homes as much choice as possible through the daily regime of the home and enhancing a sense of being in control actually prolongs life. These studies have transformed the practice of residential care.

However, this realisation only accentuates the fact that traumatising experiences may come at any point in an individual's life, and with the growth of the care home market has come a severe squeeze on the public purse to subsidise such care. The risk of care home failure is now causing considerable alarm, and the statistics on the effects of enforced care home closure paint a truly alarming picture.

We have suggested that challenging experiences may be particularly hard to cope with and so may tip over into trauma in the case of individuals who do not have the resources and requisite flexibility to adapt, accommodate and even thrive on the challenge. These are natural processes, not in themselves pathologies, but no less problematic for that.

Ageing itself is an entirely natural process, and unavoidable. As we age, and our physical capacities become reduced, the world in which we operate starts to shrink, and the once agile thought processes that we may have developed over long years become increasingly set in their ways. In terms of neural connectivity, it is perhaps on a continuum with the greater fixity of mindset that comes with trauma in early years, the more specific traumatising areas that we see in post-traumatic stress, and the debilitating effects of chronic stress.

Those older people who have a rich and active engagement show a resilience to the effects of ageing. However, when the physiological deterioration in the brain, which we know as dementia, begins to strike, the individual's capacity for managing new experiences is particularly deeply impaired and compromised. For these individuals the challenge of an enforced move would appear to be particularly stressful.

In the US, 'relocation stress syndrome' has been recognised as a nursing diagnosis since 1992, defined as *'physiologic and/or psychosocial disturbances as a result of transfer from one environment to another'*, or *'the combination of medical and psychological reactions to abrupt physical transfer that may increase the risk of grave illness or death'.*

Symptoms may include:

'... exhaustion, sleep disturbances, anxiety, grief and loss, depression and disorientation. In seniors, these symptoms are greatly exacerbated by dementia, mild cognitive impairment, poor physical health, frailty, lack of a support system, and sensory impairment. For ... seniors in particular, the resulting confusion, depression and agitation have led to increased falls, undesirable weight loss and self-care deficits.' (Greene Mintz, 2005)

The trauma of involuntary transfer, as in care home closure, is especially acute. There is good practice guidance on how to manage closures and relocations as painlessly as possible (Social Care Institute for Excellence (SCIE), 2011). Both the US and UK guidance stress maximising resident engagement and empowerment throughout the process.

However, it is still unclear how much of the devastating effect is softened by such practice – even where it is possible. Relatives Action Group for the Elderly (RAGE), which campaigns against care home closures, has argued that the ill effects of involuntary transfer cannot be eradicated. For some, at best, careful preparation under psychiatric oversight can ameliorate the risk. However, such preparation cannot be achieved for those with moderate or severe dementia because the process has to build on retained knowledge, the first of which is that the home will be closing.

According to RAGE, mortality has been roughly double the expected annual rate after involuntary care home closure. Equally worrying, if extensive consultation with residents is seen as helpful, morbidity and mortality also increase even prior to transfer, during the process of consultation.

Perhaps, then, the major implications for preventing trauma in later life, and especially the trauma of care home closure, will lie not in improved casework practice (managing individual's care and transitions) but in improved commissioning, to prevent such precipitate closures. The SCIE guidance in particular devotes a lengthy section to the ways in which care home closure may reflect 'market failure' as much as any failing in the home itself:

'Market failure occurs when the current supply is no longer able to meet demand and can be caused by a variety of economic and environmental factors. Chief among these relate to occupancy levels and the price paid for care. All providers operate within certain margins and if occupancy levels fall below a level, and therefore when income is insufficient to meet outgoing expenditure, those businesses are vulnerable to collapse ... The commissioner has a responsibility to try to understand these pressures and to ensure that no behaviour of a major purchaser such as the local commissioning authority, jeopardises the stability and viability of local business.' (SCIE, 2011)

With mounting pressure on the resources of local authorities to manage their responsibilities in provision of social care, the increasing vulnerability of the frail elderly is matched by the vulnerability of the market model for care services (Department of Health, 2009b). Were it not for other, more creative developments, the growing crisis in personal care services might then round off in grim irony this exploration of the extent to which social pressures and supports compound individuals' vulnerability to additional trauma.

Design for older living

Another key lesson is that we must reduce our reliance on residential care, and redouble efforts to maintain vulnerable people as far as possible in their own homes and in environments where they can exercise most control over their lives. Modern technology combined with modern psychology can enhance the ability of older people to remain in the homes they know, where they are most able to remain active and engaged in day-to-day pursuits.

The development of 'telecare' (electronic monitoring and communications in the home) enables practical help to be provided at home that was previously only possible in specialised units such as care homes or sheltered complexes. Linking a number of homes with a staff team based at a local complex is a very economical way to manage out-of-hours support, as well as encouraging social contact by day through social events and other welfare supports.

Another promising development is the use of the psychology and neuroscience of ageing to redesign the home environment to accommodate fading faculties, such as sight and memory, with brighter lights, careful use of colour and pattern, and labelling cupboards. A further area of interest in the psychology of enabling environments for older persons is the growth of retro-fitting (Chaplin, 2011) – the deliberate use of the wallpapers and furnishings of a previous era to strengthen the sense of being at home in a world that is fast changing, by keeping the home itself full of memories.

All of these developments in care for older people are further attempts to adjust an environment in order to promote independence and reduce the risk of events threatening to overwhelm the capacity of individuals to cope.

Nevertheless, care for the elderly is not simply care at home – there can be a community dimension too. A Memory Cafe is a place where people with dementia and their carers can meet, offering social interaction and time out from home. Moreover, they also offer activities that can have a positive effect on dementia. As parts of the brain begin to degenerate, other less used parts nevertheless remain open to new experience. Memory cafes seek to offer new stimuli in order to open these other areas of the brain, such as providing objects designed to stimulate the senses – touch, smell and taste.

There is growing evidence for the effectiveness of creative activities such as painting, writing, drawing and singing – play, in other words – in improving cognitive processes, and this is especially significant with dementia. Such activities help sufferers to keep their memories for longer, and this has a continuing beneficial impact on practical activities. They can also help informal carers develop a toolkit of experiences that they can take home and use.

These activities can then help to draw out conversation and social interaction, and encourage sufferers to reminisce. The social environment also adds the possibility for sufferers – and carers – to express their fears and frustrations, their hopes and aspirations, for ways to deal with the cognitive deficits that dementia brings, and gain strength from each other. Whereas retro-fitting might be seen initially as a form of prosthetic environment, the memory cafes show that there is also an active, constructive component to engagement with activities and with others. This does not merely compensate for fading abilities, but promotes well-being. Here too we can see the recognition of plasticity leading to new interventions, based on a more social neuroscience.

Chapter 20

Common threads

Robin Johnson

What then can we learn from the examples in this section, and from the comparisons between them? What can they tell us about common themes in effective practice? And what lessons might we learn about the nature of trauma, and especially of compound or complex trauma?

These examples come from a range of services that operate largely – but not exclusively – outside of specialist clinical settings, and that are developing new practices to work with the difficulties that underlie the problems they encounter. They are a selection of what we are calling 'social practices', for want of a more commonly accepted term for all the activities that work towards social goals and to improve the lives of others.

Nevertheless, any sample needs some kind of justification. This is, in research terms, a purposive sample with the selection criteria being that all of these accounts, in their way, shed new light on the nature of trauma, and especially on the relationship between trauma and social practice, as we have defined it. There are, in truth, many other examples that we could have chosen, but a few must serve to highlight the themes.

A common feature of most, if not all, of these examples is that they do not necessarily focus on trauma as such, but rather on one or more of its manifestations as embedded behavioural problems, appearing possibly much later in life. Only the fire service example in Chapter 13 is explicitly focused on trauma – though the Combat Stress helpline comes very close, and the older persons' closure guidance deals with transition trauma in all but name.

This is quite deliberate. We have argued that personality disorder (PD) or complex trauma in particular is best seen not solely as a result of traumatic experiences very early in life, but rather of the compounding of one negative experience or relationship upon another, repeatedly throughout life. If so, then intervention at any stage is prevention, even many years into the pathways of disruptive behaviour, distrust and mutual alienation.

The after-effects of trauma – of neglect as well as abuse – may often lie hidden under other more superficial expressions that grab the attention of those whose task is to work on some particular problem, not necessarily to see its roots. The fact that so many do intuitively recognise the underlying emotional issues is a tribute to ordinary empathy, and the wish to reach even those who have learned from experience to put up barriers in the way of trusting others.

Another striking feature of many of the practice examples we have selected here is that they had found a particular idea, technique or issue that for them has articulated or galvanised a wider concern to reach out to and engage the individuals whom they seek to work with.

It may be a broad approach, such as playwork, or Asset-Based Community Development, or the therapeutic community. It may be a more specific aspect, such as the use of profile books, the TimeBank idea, the formal turn-taking structures of a debating society, or the entanglements of the Drama Triangle. Or it may be something more abstract still, more conceptual, such as negative capability, recovery, social systems analysis, or the idea of a PIE.

In fact, it is our hope that the concept of complex trauma, as an alternative to the term personality disorder, is itself a concept that helps re-focus our thinking on what we are actually dealing with in a way that liberates the imagination and stimulates the empathy that we need to manage such problems more effectively. This is the very opposite of the melodramatic demonising of PD.

A third striking common feature – again, not in all examples, but in many – is the importance of the environment. In many cases there have been changes to the actual physical or built environment of the service. These may sometimes be small but significant, such as checking the positioning of a table by a door to allow freedom of movement and self-expression for nursery children, or simply changing the positioning of a reception area, which has been shown to reduce the incidence of assaults on staff (Intelligent Space, 2003). In other cases, careful thought to the positioning of notice boards and other instructions can make a huge difference in dispelling the feel of an institution and creating the sense of being at home.

In others, rethinking the use of the building or location of the service within it can have an impact. In the case of recovery communities, the use of an ordinary cafe rather than a designated group room in a specialist treatment unit speaks volumes for the underlying message that recovery comes from being part of a community (National Social Inclusion Programme, 2009). In the case of Victim Contact, offering support in the individual's own home makes a fundamental shift in the emotional message of the service.

However, in most of the instances quoted here, it is changes in the social environment, the matrix of relationships, the social structure of roles and the opportunities for active social engagement that have been either the central focus or the key by-product of the intervention. The significance of changes in the built environment is almost entirely tied up with the impact those changes will have on the psychological and social environment, and the personal encounters, the wealth of new learning opportunities or past memories, that this creates.

Even so, perhaps the most constant recurring theme in the social engagement aspect of the enabling environment – a term we will return to – is the importance of relationships with peers. While the relationships between staff and users are important, it is often crucially in the relationships between peers that the most valuable resource lies.

Other threads

There are three or four other issues that seem to interweave through many of these accounts, which may not only indicate the direction that constructive practice tends to take, but also suggest the connection between effective practice and the underlying issues that practice is responding to (Johnson, 1981).

First, there are issues of 'personalisation' and user-led services, offering greater choice, involvement and control of their service to users. From the child-led philosophy of playwork to the nursery profile books, from individual assertiveness to psychotherapy, from TimeBanks to the person-centred planning and support for reminiscence in dementia care, the need for approaches and services of all kinds to reach out to the individual and empower them seems especially relevant when working with individuals who have been radically undermined by trauma or are at renewed risk.

Personalisation is sometimes presented as primarily an economic issue – the idea that giving choice over services helps ensure that each service user can pick and choose and get more or less the services that are right for them, customised and therefore most efficient to meet their particular needs. However, the evidence of practice suggests that for those who are most vulnerable, and especially for those for whom past trauma creates difficulties in relationships, the real value of personalisation may lie as much in the restoring of a sense of self-directedness.

The second closely related issue is that of making space for creativity, or the 'negative capability' that Brown and Webb referred to. Opportunities for creativity are perhaps the simplest way to create, in practice, the empowering and individualising atmosphere that allows individuals to take control of their own lives.

While from a straightforward point of view this may seem like a good thing, it actually runs directly counter to the increasing tendency in contemporary commissioning to measure a service's 'added value' by how well it reaches specified 'outcomes'. For services working with those who have experienced trauma, perhaps, there will be a need for greater creativity on the part of commissioners, and on the part of service providers, to show what they have really achieved.

The third theme that appears in so many of these accounts is the importance of working with people's aspirations, ambitions and hopes. This emphasis on goals and motivations – the counterpart to creativity – is typical of the more humanistic tradition in psychology, which is explored a little further in the discussions in Section three. Here we may simply note that it is the direct opposite of seeing vulnerable individuals as being defined by their vulnerability, let alone being seen as trapped in a neurology that claims to 'explain' how and who they are.

The more self-confident and assertive will arguably be well able to focus on their goals and strengths for themselves. However, for those who have been marginalised and traumatised, special efforts to reach out and engage may be necessary. As Rex Haigh has argued, those who are diagnosed with PD have commonly been in abusive and asymmetrical relationships where others have abused their power and done horrible things to them, and they will therefore be exquisitely sensitive to this being repeated by services that are not really listening to them.

Of course, most such issues are now seen as good practice throughout many areas of service provision and social practice. However the frequency with which they appear in these accounts hints at the possibility that these concerns may be especially significant for services working with those who have suffered abuse or neglect in the past.

How far it may be true that past trauma, and the pervasive malaise and loss of security in the world that trauma brings, underlies many failures to use services well, and the need for services to adjust accordingly, needs to be better understood. This will clearly be a key area for future research. However, research here does not only mean having researchers coming to visit a service, observe, record, and go away. The need for all staff to be pro-actively involved in asking the right questions about their practice is clear.

A further theme that appears in many of these accounts is summed up by the phrase 'reflective practice'. All the narratives here give some account of thinking through the way that a service used to operate, questioning whether things need to be done in the same way, and arriving at ideas for change in the ways the service might operate. In many cases, that process is shared, collective and owned by all the staff of a service. In some cases, that rethinking extends to involve service users.

Where that process starts with the emotional aspects of working in a challenging environment, we may hope to see a more supportive, robust and yet tolerant unit culture. Where the process starts with an idea, or a research finding, we may hope to see a contribution to the process of research itself. In this way, we reach our way, as a society, towards the development of more 'psychologically informed' or 'enabling' environments. These are ideas that we will now explore further, in more practical detail, in the final section of this book.

Finally, these services and initiatives have been by their nature both holistic (they take the whole situation and work with it) and humanistic (they take the whole person, and work with them). It would be impossible to do justice to the examples given here by reducing what they have each done to some kind of formula, or boiling down all these elements in their subtle ecology of care to a few supposed 'active ingredients' that can then be extrapolated, replicated and measured, as a way to find the 'real' evidence of their effectiveness.

Section three

The future

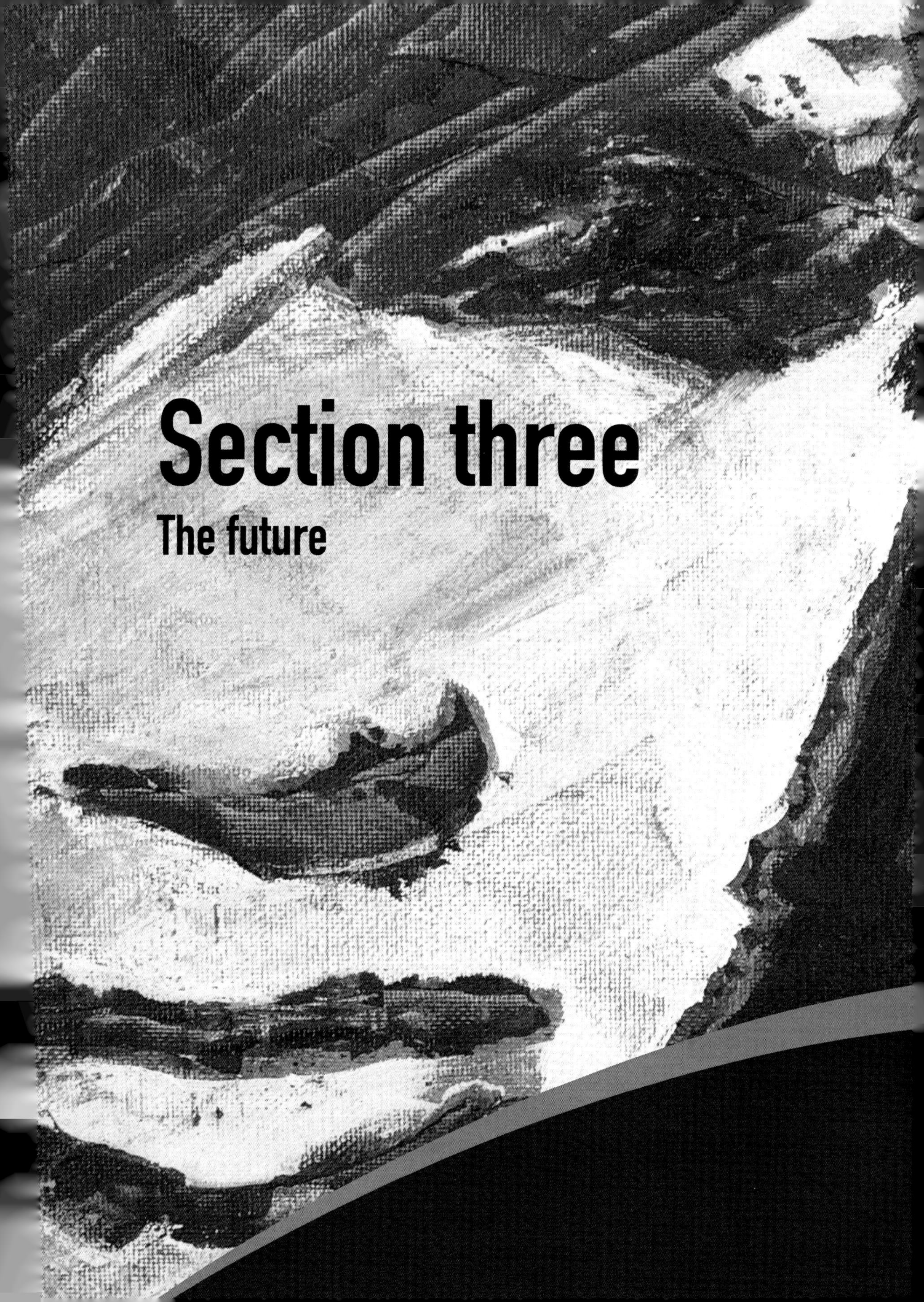

Section three:

The future

Introduction

The third and final section of this book looks to the future and explores developments in policy, research and practice that seem to chart a new path, or a multiplicity of paths, towards a world in which lived experience, social values, emotional intelligence, relational health and the crucial element of social connectedness between people are given their full due.

In our overview of psychological problems in homelessness, we suggested that the best use of specialist psychological or psychotherapeutic expertise is not to create new referral mechanisms for new health services, but to develop a role for specialist expertise working with other, non-mental health services to develop the capacity to manage mental health problems they encounter together. We will return to the newly forming alliance between specialist and non-specialist services that we see coming into being.

In the examples of homelessness resettlement, what comes over most frequently is the importance and the role of the whole environment – both the built environment and the social world – to complement and supplement the skills and emotional intelligence of staff. An individual's skills are important, certainly, but the reinforcement of the group as a whole and the organisational culture of a service are equally critical. We will then consider a new approach to services for the more vulnerable, the marginalised and excluded, via carefully developed psychologically informed environments.

We will then outline some new approaches to the creation of more enlightened and 'enabling' practice, in the social environments in which we aim to live and grow. We go on to look at a similar attempt to enhance the ways that whole societies, and specific businesses, services and communities, are striving to become more emotionally intelligent, and to develop 'enabling environments'.

Chapter 21

Communities, once and future

Robin Johnson and Rex Haigh[1]

The concept of a psychologically informed environment (PIE) is still relatively new.

First introduced in 2010 in the journal *Mental Health and Social Inclusion*, the idea was immediately adopted by the Department for Communities and Local Government and the National Mental Health Development Unit and used in new guidance then being developed, to encourage innovative practice in homelessness resettlement work. The concept of a PIE seemed to describe the more sophisticated and thoughtful approach to resettlement that they wished to promote, in units such as hostels and refuges that were working with homeless people with sometimes severe and entrenched psychological and emotional difficulties.

The original thinking behind PIEs arose from work being undertaken under the aegis of the Royal College of Psychiatrists (RCP) to develop a new vocabulary for community mental health. This work of the RCP in turn stemmed from the attempt to refresh and revive the concept of a therapeutic community (TC) – an approach that had developed in the years immediately after the Second World War (Main, 1946).

The TC had evolved over some years into one of the few treatment modalities with any real claim to success in working with individuals with a diagnosis of personality disorder (PD), but it was struggling to articulate the successes it was seeing in the prescribed measurement styles required in an age of evidence-based medicine. The RCP development group initially set out to put the TC approach on a more sound footing for the brave new world of evidence and commissioning.

---

1 The following article has been adapted from material first published in a trilogy of papers titled 'Social psychiatry and social policy for the 21st century', in *Mental Health and Social Inclusion* **14** (4) 30–35; **15** (1) 17–23; **15** (2) 57–65.

However, it also hoped to articulate a wider aspiration than the original concept of a TC could cover. The TC as a model, it was feared, had by then become identified with a particular way of working that now seemed too narrow and specialist to embody the emerging vision of the place of psychological and psychotherapeutic thinking in the contemporary world.

The intention was to stimulate new thinking in what was being called 'the new social psychiatry' to face the challenges of a new century. This is an era marked by growing concern for the mental health of the population at large, and at the same time, increasing recognition of the social determinants of health. Reliance on specialist treatment services no longer seemed the only way forward for community mental health.

In this chapter we will attempt to:

- outline the origins and early evolution of the TC as a model
- explore the contribution that TC thinking made to the development of progressive practice, first in mental health and later in social policy more broadly
- outline the internal debates over the direction of the TC approach, and the ways in which it found itself sidelined when other new approaches emerged, including the widespread use of new psychotropic medications.

The TC and the early evolution of social psychiatry

The idea of a therapeutic community – a place and a way of living about which people could say, 'living here is the treatment' – has a very long history. It can be glimpsed, for example, in the principles of respect and moral (or more accurately, 'morale') treatment as originally developed at the York Retreat, the psychiatric community created by the Quakers in 1796 (Stewart, 1992). In the Quaker community's insistence on respect for all, we can see with hindsight one of the earliest expressions of a values-led and person-centred approach, which now seems remarkably modern.

However, the more immediate origins of the TC, as a mental health treatment model, go back to the Second World War, with a small group of psychoanalysts enlisted into the British Army who were concerned to learn the lessons of the failed treatments of shell shock in the First World War. Armed with new concepts that aimed to uncover the hidden roots of psychiatric symptoms, they began to run their army hospital units in a new, distinctly experimental and quite radical fashion (Trist & Murray, 1990; Harrison, 1999).

They started by replacing conventional treatment with lectures and discussion on the meaning of symptoms, day-to-day life and problem-solving. In the place of conventional and strict hospital routine, which encouraged patients to be passive recipients of professional care, they substituted a more open discussion about what was happening and what was and what was not helpful towards patients' recovery. Patients were encouraged to do things for themselves, to get involved in the running of the units, even to disagree with the care staff and give their own views on their own and each other's experiences.

It is perhaps hardly surprising that some of these experiments quickly ran afoul of the military authorities; some, indeed, lasted only a few weeks before being terminated. However, the idea of a new kind of psychiatry actively questioning the immediate social and institutional environment and supporting change was taking root – not simply as an abstract, philosophical critique, but as a programme of day-to-day hands-on practical engagement and enquiry. After the war ended, a number of specialist rehabilitation units were established to apply the learning from these early experiments in rehabilitation and resettlement work with those individuals severely traumatised by their wartime experiences, such as concentration camp survivors, and it was here that the idea of a TC was first fully formulated.

The mould

Over this period some of the key tenets of the TC 'model' were first established, articulated, and later institutionalised. In *Community as Doctor*, an influential study of the pioneering work of the Henderson hospital, the sociologist Robert Rappoport described (1960) the organisational approach that had evolved there. It consisted of a complex interlocking structure of:

- small ongoing psychotherapy groups
- various task groups for particular practical purposes
- a large daily community group for shared decision-making.

The study also first identified and articulated the core TC working principles of democratisation, permissiveness, communalism and reality-confrontation that he saw in action there, alongside a 'flattened hierarchy' in which all participants had, in principle, an equal vote – even if some views carried more weight than others.

These principles resonated with the post-war liberal democratic mood in the West, where more authoritarian regimes had been seen to fail. This radically democratised model of a hospital soon became archetypal, the standard architecture of such treatment units in psychiatric settings. Gradually they began to be seen as the template for 'proper' TCs everywhere.

Yet even alongside this gradual standardisation of the basic TC model there were calls – especially from some of the founding fathers of the new movement – to retain a more open, constantly evolving approach. Tom Main, who had first suggested the term 'therapeutic community' based on his work at the Cassel Hospital, argued for what he called a *'culture of enquiry'*, in which all actions and all structures need to be open to fresh scrutiny and discussion.

Maxwell Jones, the founder of the Henderson Hospital, was by then working not in an isolated specialist treatment unit, but in an ordinary catchment area hospital covering three rural counties of Scotland. Here, he introduced the notion of living/learning (Jones, 1968) as a conscious attempt to move away from exclusively relying on the terminology of therapy, in the hope to encourage the idea that all participants in a community, both staff and patients, families and ordinary citizens, all need to be 'on a learning curve'.

There were also several notable attempts to develop TC approaches in prisons – another area of considerable financial and symbolic investment for the management of many highly troubled individuals. Here, it was important to find an effective way to reconcile society's somewhat contradictory wishes to protect the public by containing the offender and punishing them for their misdeeds, while at the same time reducing the likelihood of future offending by rehabilitating them.

For some years, these early experiments in 'social therapy' seemed to hold out the best hopes for the future of psychiatry. They offered an exciting, progressive option for remodelling the hospital itself into a more therapeutic environment. Psychotherapy and the hospital milieu would not merely co-exist, they would inform and learn from each other. In 1953, for example, the World Health Organization was able to say:

'... the more the psychiatric hospital imitates the general hospital as it at present exists, the less successful it will be in creating the atmosphere it needs. Too many psychiatric hospitals give the impression of being an uneasy compromise between a general hospital and a prison. Whereas ... the creation of the atmosphere of a therapeutic community is in itself one of the most important types of treatment which the psychiatric hospital can provide.'

A movement sideways

There were, however, other new developments being explored that had a profound effect on the future of TCs. New medications offered the promise of a less challenging and time-consuming means to empty the old Victorian hospitals and rapidly return people to the community. First synthesised in 1950, chlorpromazine – 'Largactil' – brought the promise of a 'magic bullet' for psychosis, and was in widespread use by the end of the 1950s. Antidepressants and the 'minor' tranquillisers – 'mother's little helper', as they were rather sardonically named – soon followed. Great claims were made for the effectiveness of these treatments, now rather less in evidence (Moncrieff, 2007). For some years, the apparent success of the new psychotropic medications seemed to offer a more immediate hope for a cure, and certainly one that seemed less disruptive to hospital life and routines.

As new generations of powerful and effective psychotropics were developed, the old division between a psychotherapeutic and a biomedical approach to treatment became ever more stark. As a result, social psychiatry, which worked primarily with understanding personal meanings, relationships and context, was relegated to a more specialist role in psychotherapy or in supportive counselling, and the early promise and early growth of TCs in the UK and elsewhere has not been sustained, at least within mainstream healthcare. Gradually, the TC approach within the NHS became restricted to a small number of specialist units, with a more specialist focus, reserved for more complex and intractable problems such as the treatment of PD (Vaglum *et al*, 1982). More recently, even many of these have been forced to close.

There was, however, one positive: the founding principles and the practice of the TC had been established.

Yet from the start there had been debates and disagreements about what should count as the most fundamental principles of a TC, their essential core or the 'active ingredient'. There were ongoing and lively debates within the TC movement over, for example, the nature of democracy and authority, the double-edged role of charismatic leadership, the possible role of individual therapy alongside group work, the usefulness or otherwise of psychoanalytic interpretation, the nature of sanctions in reality confrontation, the significance of boundaries and many other such issues (Hinshelwood & Manning, 1979).

Other communities, other needs

The most obvious dissenters within the ranks of the TC movement were those units established to deal with the growing problems of substance abuse. In 1958, a quite different form of the TC emerged from Alcoholics Anonymous groups in New York, when Chuck Dederich formed Synanon. This was the beginning of what came to be known as 'concept-based', 'hierarchical', 'behavioural' or 'programmatic' TCs. More recently they have tended to be known as 'addiction communities', since this is the population and need for which this structure seems most suited. Worldwide, this is a movement that now comprises tens of thousands of units, with variable degrees of adherence to the original Synanon model, but all of which style themselves as 'therapeutic communities'.

In the early addiction TCs, the permissiveness of the British model was replaced by strict adherence to a behavioural code (most obviously in abstinence). Highly confrontative encounter groups took the place of the reflective psychotherapeutic small groups, and a clear hierarchy of command emerged, with graduates of the programme in charge of enforcement of rules and sanctions, rather than the democratic government by the community as a whole. This initially seems a very different kind of entity. However, the common threads have been increasingly recognised (Haigh & Lees, 2008), and a false polarisation into pure democratic vs pure hierarchical TCs is no longer tenable: most hierarchical TCs are more democratic than often thought, and democratic TCs are more hierarchical than is often thought.

In prisons, similarly, some of the key features that others had thought essential to TCs, such as the authority of the community to manage its own boundaries and membership, were simply not achievable. In the tension between the need for security and the need for therapy it is generally the requirements of security that come first. For example, economic pressures with reduced staff levels, cutting across other priorities, can restrict the number of therapy groups that can be held in a week (or they may be cancelled at short notice), and can increase 'lock-down time' during which prisoners are locked in individual cells and unable to take part in any informal therapeutic activity.

There were also difficulties in translating the central TC conceptions and model into other areas of social welfare services, such as residential children's services. Those specialist units developed during the 1930s and 40s, for those who were then called 'maladjusted' children, had developed their own community approach and vocabulary, as well as a professional association called the Planned Environment Therapy Trust (Dockar-Drysdale, 1974). Although there seemed to be many clear points of similarity between these communities' psychologically informed approach and the underlying principles and therapeutic goals of TCs, there were also some evident differences. It was not until the late 1970s that the two movements began to identify their common ground and meet to debate the nature of the variations.

New ideas of 'community'

As well as the wider developments, there were also debates over the nature of 'community' itself. How far did a community need to be separate from the world outside in order to effect real change? Could a day care centre operate as a TC, for example? There were some who argued that it could only be a watered down version of the real thing, lacking the intensity of total immersion and the 24-hour wrap-around experience (Clark, 1965). A school of thought arose that what made a community was not essentially the building but the belonging – a shared commitment, a pooled accountability, a common language or approach (Al-Khudhairy, 2000). The degree of immersion in the experience might be variable (Johnson, 1981), and the building or buildings where this happened might be little more than a practical convenience.

The idea gradually emerged of creating a dispersed but still cohesive community, a new kind of intentional community of like-minded people, mutually supportive and psychologically minded.

Another question that arose asked whether 'therapy' as such was actually the only model for personal change that was to be promoted or valued. Two new schools of thought began to propose an alternative view. With the growth of psychology both as a body of thought and as a profession, social skills models of mental health were now emerging, suggesting that a psycho-educational framework may be as or more helpful than an illness/cure model. Here at least there were clear points of connection with the special schools. However, there are also clear echoes of this in mainstream education with social and emotional aspects of learning and wider concepts of pedagogy.

Social policy moves on

In the wider sphere of social policy there was also increasing talk of a 'social model of disability', which suggested that much of the disability that disabled people encountered in their lives came primarily from society's inability to include and consider their needs. This recognition led, via the Disability Discrimination Act (1995), to a programme of negotiating 'reasonable adjustments' to the way that the ordinary agencies and services in society operate, ensuring that they do not unwittingly bring about the marginalisation of individuals who are 'at risk'.

Social inclusion can then best be described as the action agenda for the social model of disability. That is, it begins with a recognition that much of the 'disability' experienced by disabled people is arguably more a result of the way society is organised – wheelchair access being the most visible example (Oliver, 1990a; 1990b; Sayce, 2000). However, social inclusion work goes rather further than the law in attempting to promote a more positive attitude towards those at risk of exclusion. Social inclusion policies (Social Exclusion Unit, 2004; National Social Inclusion Programme, 2009) now encourage all services in the broader community to be more conscious of the mental health and emotional needs of those at risk of marginalisation.

For the TC movement, perhaps the most obvious significance in the social model of disability was that it prompted a reconsideration of the links with those residential communities that were established for people with a learning difficulty. These were certainly communities, but they were setting out to shelter and empower, not to change. There is no 'therapy' if there is no illness to cure. However, social inclusion policies, focusing on the interface between the individual and the community, have challenged society's habitual reliance on separate services for those with more challenging needs, and this challenge extends to questioning the need for specialist care homes or sheltered housing for those with learning difficulties, for example.

Whether in secluded specialist communities, or in the community 'at large', suddenly the language of the TC risked alienating and marginalising a whole population of vulnerable people already disenfranchised in too many ways. Was this still the conception that could carry the ambition for a more engaged and a more social psychiatry?

While formal TCs may have been on the retreat in the UK health service, therefore, many of the principles and values that the early TC pioneers espoused – such as 'user' involvement and empowerment, greater flexibility and responsiveness in services, transparency and accountability of the professionals – have passed into the mainstream of UK social policy. Meanwhile, many of the underlying ideas and much of the terminology were taken up with some enthusiasm outside the hospital system, in day care centres and in residential care homes for rehabilitation (Janssen, 1980).

With the dawning of the 21st century, new considerations were emerging along with new catalysts for change.

PD and the challenge to 'therapeutic nihilism'

One key driver for that change, which had a profound effect on the future of TCs, was the growing demand for NHS mental health services to include the needs of a range of people with evident mental health problems, such as those with PDs, whom mental health services until then had been reluctant to take on. Attempts were made to confront the 'therapeutic nihilism' that claimed that such problems were formally untreatable (at least in a narrow clinical sense) and therefore could not be the responsibility of treatment agencies, as psychiatric services now saw themselves.

In 2004, the Department of Health, via one of its spin-off organisations, the National Institute for Mental Health in England (NIMHE), issued a document (Department of Health, 2004) declaring in forthright terms that PD was to be *'no longer a diagnosis of exclusion'* – that is, a diagnosis that could be used to deny sufferers access to secondary mental health services on the grounds of their supposed 'untreatability'.

The new policy came with modest funding attached to establish a number of pilots in various parts of the country over which NIMHE would take the lead. These pilots were to explore and demonstrate what could be achieved by the creation of new and experimental services to work specifically with people with PD. In line with the spirit of the age – and with the experience of those clinicians who had worked with the PD group – these services were to have extensive and in-depth 'user involvement'.

Not unconnected here were the mounting calls to find a better solution to the worryingly high numbers of people in the prison population found to have significant mental health problems. These needs went largely untreated and, particularly when linked – as they so often were – with self-medication via substance abuse, were thought to be in part responsible for a cycle of alienation and re-offending that was proving hard to break. The costs to society as a whole of not managing these issues, or of managing them only within a custodial/punitive framework, were becoming evident. Where deterrence fails, treatment must step in.

One treatment modality that did have some claim to success with this population, and an evidence base to support it, was the TC (Lees, 2004). However, if this was now to be brought in from the cold and promoted to motivate, inform and guide new treatment services, the endless debates around what was and what was not a TC, or what exactly it was that worked in a TC approach, would need to be resolved. The NHS, increasingly wedded to 'evidence-based treatments', had a marked preference for random controlled trials and for large numbers in order to gather sufficient statistical power and significance. The TC simply did not produce this kind of evidence, but there was some concern now to review the evidence, such as it was, and to justify the claims for the efficacy of TCs.

This new concern began with the return of calls for some degree of standardisation, at least in the definition of the overarching model. Accordingly, in the UK context, for example, the RCP self-regulation wing, the Centre for Quality Improvement, agreed to convene a series of discussions and meetings (which came to be called the Community of Communities) to attempt to find or devise a set of core standards that UK TCs might all adhere to, including a framework for recognising the different modalities of therapy and community that might be seen as legitimate variants on the key themes. We will return to these efforts later.

Another world outside of health and social care

Seemingly quite unconnected with this health service evolution, a wholly new kind of welfare service was being established through the peculiarities of the social security benefits system in the UK, offering what was termed 'housing-related support' to people either homeless or at high risk of becoming homeless, or of going into more institutional care. A range of services were being developed to assist vulnerable people in living with greater independence, in ordinary, non-institutional housing.

Such services and the essential funding to support them could then be available without regard to the individual's particular vulnerability, diagnosis or category of care service. It was based simply on the day-to-day practical needs of the vulnerable, not on any specialist clinical assessment or criteria. It was a model that fitted perfectly the non-labelling of the social inclusion theme. There was in consequence a rapid growth in such support services, including for many who would not be eligible or suitable for mainstream mental health care. Such services began to respond to and cater for the problems of PD and traumatised, chaotic lives that the mental health services had been overlooking.

In accordance with the prevailing zeitgeist, such housing-based support services increasingly stressed the importance of individually focused support. In practice, however, the majority of services had their roots in specialist housing services such as hostels, refuges and warden-aided supported accommodation, where, as one sheltered accommodation manager put it, *'This is not just a building with services in it; this is a whole community'.*

Significantly, the value of 'peer support' in such supportive housing services was also formally recognised. Facilitating positive interactions between residents was actually seen as something that could quite properly be funded and supported by housing services, as part of their own service. Sometimes consciously borrowed, sometimes freshly reinvented, some of the underlying themes that the TC movement had articulated were reappearing in a new guise. Despite, or perhaps precisely because of, the official stress on individual outcomes, there was clearly a need for some new kind of language to describe what else was going on in these community settings that captured the nature of supportive relationships, a sense of common purpose and of belonging, and the establishment of an emotionally safe and supportive environment that for many people was proving pivotal to successful recovery, or to a sustained quality of life.

It became clear, for example, that a homelessness hostel was not merely a conveyor belt operation, processing individuals and moving them on. It was not simply a place to live after a time on the streets, but a crucial environment in which individuals, with the support of others, could re-examine their lives, break old habits, relearn ways. The idea emerged that hostels had to be seen as 'places for change'. This implies some kind of 'remedial' impetus, but one that is outside the health service, and well outside the territory that is normally described as 'therapeutic'. Yet it represents the idea of a supportive community as the agent for resettlement and reintegration into mainstream life.

The concept of a psychologically aware or 'psychologically informed' environment was partly a simple attempt to describe some of the more innovative services developing in this field. However, it was also a quite deliberate attempt to avoid simply re-triggering the familiar discussion of what could constitute a TC. In particular, it was important to encourage frontline staff and service users to rely more on their own experience, and find their own solutions as to 'how we might do things differently'. By creating a new term, the intention was to stimulate fresh discussion – to rewind the clock and start with the culture of enquiry, rather than recycling the Rappoport model.

There was no intention to renounce the long history and tradition of the TC, but outside the mindset of the TC there were clearly an increasing number of inventive and innovative programmes in areas such as youth and community work, in occupational health, in prevention, and especially in supported housing and homelessness services. In other areas of 'ordinary life', too, there is now a string of studies confirming the importance of suitable work for allowing people a sense of inclusion, purpose and value.

Public health and social cohesion

The increasing sophistication and cost of biomedical interventions to save and improve life have extended life expectancy, but success in terms of general mental health, satisfaction with life, personal fulfilment and happiness of the population has declined. Not just in the UK but throughout the developed world the level of prescriptions for depression and for stress-related conditions has grown exponentially.

There is also increasing concern at the role and cost of workplace stress, especially as teamwork skills replace physical strength in the increasingly knowledge-based and service-focused economy. With the increasing assertiveness of health and safety legislation, there is a growing recognition that the employer's duty of care towards the workforce extends to a concern for workplace mental health for all, and not simply for those who are most vulnerable.

While the total cost to the economy of days lost oweing to sickness has been calculated, the reduction in productivity due to poor staff morale and through management time absorbed in resolving internal conflicts remains incalculable. Meanwhile, positive workforce ambitions, as expressed in such programmes as Investors in People suggest that engagement is the key to maximum productivity.

This has led to growing interest in the wider sphere of preventive health, the social context and the social determinants of health, and public mental health. With sickness and absenteeism in the workplace growing, with our prisons filling with people with mental health, drug and alcohol problems, the idea that the health service looked after our health, the economy our income, and the prison systems dealt with crime, became simply untenable.

In the UK, this heralded the era of 'joined up government' – the recognition that, at a national level, policy initiatives and performance measurements needed to support each other and not blindly create gaps in the welfare net, while at local level the relevant services need to be working together. In particular, a new ambition began to arise for a more proactive approach to prevention and public health. Not merely in health promotion campaigns – smoking cessation etc – but in active engagement with the 'social determinants of health'.

The extent of this sea change away from a simple medical framework for understanding community mental health is summarised concisely in the Young Foundations' summary report, *Sinking and swimming: Understanding Britain's Unmet Needs* (2009). Nor is this rethink confined to the UK or the particularly aggressive depredations of social and community spirit wrought by the so-called Anglo-Saxon economic model. In their introduction to the World Health Organization's study (2003) of the social determinants of health, epidemiologists Wilkinson and Marmot state:

'Health policy was once thought to be about little more than the provision and funding of medical care … [But] while medical care can prolong survival and improve prognosis … more important for the health of the population as a whole are the social and economic conditions that make people ill…

*[H]owever important **individual** genetic susceptibilities to disease may be, the common causes of the ill health that affects **populations** are environmental: they come and go far more quickly than the slow pace of genetic change because they reflect the changes in the way we live.*

... much depends on understanding the interaction between material disadvantage and its social meanings. It is not simply that poor material circumstances are harmful to health; the social meaning of being poor, unemployed, socially excluded, or otherwise stigmatized also matters. As social beings, we need not only good material conditions but ... to feel valued and appreciated. We need friends, we need more sociable societies, we need to feel useful, and we need to exercise a significant degree of control over meaningful work. Without these we become more prone to depression, drug use, anxiety, hostility and feelings of hopelessness, which all rebound on physical health.' (Marmot & Wilkinson, 2003)

We are seeing increasing recognition of the wider social context of health, mental health and well-being (Marmot & Wilkinson, 2003; Young Foundations, 2009; Royal College of Psychiatrists, 2010). There is also a growing concern for public health and prevention, with the common mental health problems of depression and anxiety, PDs, substance abuse and other, sometimes subtler forms of self-harm, now seen as lying at the heart of these efforts (Department of Health, 2010; Milton, 2010).

The once and future community

With the roll out of the Department of Health's PD pilots, we are also seeing something of a revival of services explicitly calling themselves TCs (although some use the name with caution and hide it behind phrases such as 'complex needs services' on their official websites). 2011 saw the creation of a new umbrella organisation, The Community of Therapeutic Communities (TCTC). This will be a new incorporated UK charity, which aims to join together and advance the work undertaken by professional organisations – both with adults (Association of Therapeutic Communities) and with children (Charterhouse Group).

Clearly the extraordinary dynamism and transformative power of the original TC model in specialist treatment units has not gone away. Yet it is no longer the only yardstick for positive engagement that has a psycho-social or a community dimension. We have, in addition, the PIEs movement in homelessness, and the psychologically informed planned environments in the prison service, as outlined in Chapter 1.

It now becomes both necessary and possible to explore a wider range of issues that impact upon individual and community well-being. However, for this we must go beyond the notion of a planned or specialist treatment environment, and we will need to introduce a further, and considerably broader, concept – the 'enabling environment'.

To sum up: as we move further into the 21st century, we not only face new challenges in the development of a broader social psychiatry that is suited to its times, but we are also presented with new opportunities. In this new climate, fresh ideas are emerging that attempt to provide a vocabulary for the community approach to mental health, and the mental health approach to public health, that was previously lacking.

The following chapters aim to set out a number of new ideas that are attempting to explore the central importance of the social dimensions of health and the healthcare impacts of everyday life and practice for individual and community well-being. These new concepts aim both to embody current new thinking and to encourage new practice.

Either way, it will be the recognition of the significance of relationships and relatedness (Puttnam, 2000; Christakis & Fowler, 2009; Norman, 2010) that is central to any efforts to enhance mental health and improve the health of the nation.

This is the real foundation of 'the new social psychiatry'.

Chapter 22

Psychology in the environment

Robin Johnson and Rex Haigh[1]

'... the definitive marker of a PIE is simply that, if asked why the unit is run in such and such a way, the staff would give an answer couched in terms of the emotional and psychological needs of the service users, rather than giving a logistical or practical rationale, such as convenience, costs, or health and safety regulations.'

The 'psychologically informed environment'

In July 2010, the Department for Communities and Local Government (CLG), in conjunction with the National Mental Health Development Unit (NMHDU), published new guidance on better ways of meeting the psychological and emotional needs of people who are homeless that was aimed at frontline homelessness resettlement services, and for those who commission such services (CLG/NMHDU, 2010).

The guidance stressed the need for services to recognise that many of their clientele will have suffered some degree of emotional trauma, and the need to be able to respond appropriately.

Citing and promoting a string of examples of innovative practice, it then in summary introduced a new term to the vocabulary of service provision – that of the psychologically informed environment (PIE). The aim of the PIE approach is to recognise, endorse and encourage more of such enlightened work in hostels, refuges etc.

---

1 The following article has been adapted from material first published in a trilogy of papers titled 'Social psychiatry and social policy for the 21st century', in *Mental Health and Social Inclusion* **14** (4) 30–35; **15** (1) 17–23; **15** (2) 57–65.

For example, we expect a prison to have high walls, security gates and cameras; or a hostel to have a reception area, bedspaces, perhaps a communal lounge and possibly a training kitchen. However, when in addition the task of the service is the treatment, rehabilitation or any other form of management of problematic behaviour, we need to ask how well the environment is designed to meet the psychological and emotional needs of its population. The guidance suggested that, wherever any agency has effective control over many aspects of the day-to-day lives of the individuals living there (such as in a hostel, a hospital or a prison), we have in effect a highly managed environment. We therefore have an environment that is, or can be, consciously planned for the purpose of personal change to some degree.

There will inevitably be practical constraints, but with some thought, any environment – both the physical and the social environment of rules and expectations – may be adapted as far as possible to enhance this aspect of the work. The concept of a PIE then describes any service that consciously attempts to identify, adapt and use all available aspects of the environment, the resources and the day-to-day functioning of the service, to focus on addressing the psychological needs and emotional issues thrown up by the residents.

Action learning and service evolution

As to how any one service may approach the task in practice, the field is entirely open. In essence, wherever psychological considerations of any kind can be translated meaningfully into carefully redesigning and managing the social environment, then we have a PIE. It is these practical changes in day-to-day running, in the use of space etc, that define a PIE.

For the moment, at least, the definitive marker of a PIE is simply that, if asked why the unit is run in such and such a way, the staff would give an answer couched in terms of the emotional and psychological needs of the service users, rather than giving a logistical or practical rationale, such as convenience, costs, or health and safety regulations.

However, the key to psychological thinking here is not imbibing received wisdom, or even acquiring new therapeutic skills, but reflective practice. Although staff training may well help, the CLG guidance stresses the central role of shared and thoughtful learning from experience:

'[R]eflective practice is advantageous in three distinct ways:

- *Firstly, by aiming to recognise and understand service users' difficulties, it helps to generate among clients a sense of being understood and 'heard'. It enables keyworkers to identify and defuse potential conflicts, and so to ensure safe practice.*
- *Secondly, it enables staff to get some perspective on the emotional challenges in their work, thereby enabling some distance from it and the possibility of working out the emotional content of the work being done. In this way anxieties may be reduced and burnout may also go down.*
- *Thirdly, it enables shared learning cycles to be set up which enhance the acquisition of skills. Staff attending such groups have the opportunity to discuss the models and techniques employed to facilitate change in detail, and corrective feedback may be offered.'* (CLG/NMHDU, 2010)

The guidance goes on to note: *'Recent evidence has indicated that negative beliefs about the population reduced and perceptions of effective working increased, in addition to burnout falling, when a programme of reflective practice group work was added to a training course.'*

It then observes dryly that: *'There are obvious time and cost commitments involved in enabling front-line staff to attend regular supervision, typically for an hour and a half every two weeks. It is vital therefore that managers 'buy in' to the concept and are able to perceive the benefits in order that a long-term commitment can be made.'*

This clearly also requires an enlightened attitude in local commissioning of the service that allows the time and scope for frontline staff to think, discuss and argue over how things could perhaps be done differently, and make whatever suitable changes they can. The guidance is therefore aimed as much at commissioners as it is at frontline staff and managers.

Finally, we should not overlook the impact of the built environment itself. A number of studies (Cooper Marcus, 2007; Malenbaum *et al*, 2009) have demonstrated, for example, that a pleasant view of greenery in a central courtyard can delay the deterioration of mental functioning of those afflicted with dementia. Even the positioning of a reception area and security lights in a hostel can completely change the institutional atmosphere from something alienating to something welcoming (Intelligent Space, 2003). A planned environment can be planned on many levels (Lawlor & Webb, 2009).

High risk or secure environments

The PIE concept originally arose out of the need to recognise and to work with the levels of emotional trauma that accompany an individual becoming homeless, and the possibility is being explored of a more thoughtfully designed environment in residential resettlement settings, such as in homeless persons' hostels, women's refuges and foyers for homeless youths (CLG, 2006; CLG/NMHDU, 2010).

The PIE approach is focused primarily on institutions – that is, on services that have considerable control over the day-to-day lives of individuals in their care, and which need to recognise with clarity and sensitivity the psychological and emotional aspects of their work. There is no reason, however, why the same thoughtful consideration cannot be given to the design of a day care or drop-in service. However, the PIE concept seems in principle to have a potentially wider applicability, beyond hostels and refuges and such places, and can apply to any services attempting to manage marginalised groups more effectively, with greater thought.

In the context of the prison service, for example, the concept of a psychologically informed and carefully planned environment may in many situations be more useful than the earlier notion of a therapeutic community (TC), at least as it is commonly defined. However, there are clearly other successful and constructive prison and youth offender institutions that are not TCs as such, but which, in some perhaps less clearly articulated way, do manage to create and use positive relationships very effectively. Here, too, we may now need to find another vocabulary and another set of key principles to describe what is most effective in the most constructive prison regimes, and also, for example, in approved premises (formerly known as 'probation hostels').

In homelessness resettlement, such changes may come about gradually and incrementally. In a more controlled environment such as a prison, where all changes in the daily routine must be thoroughly managed in great detail, introducing a PIE may need to be more tightly planned. Here we need to think more in terms of planned change – a psychologically informed *planned* environment (PIPE) – and there are currently discussions within the National Offender Management Service over the nature of the changes that might be introduced in several pilots over then next year or more. The common thread, however, is that these changes come about through the application of careful approaches to the psychological and emotional needs – and potential – of the residents.

Variety and ecological 'fit'

With the notion of a PIE, there is no assumption at all that structured group work, democratic decision-making, communalism, permissive self-expression, reality-confrontation, or any of the features commonly associated with the archetypal TC model (Rappoport, 1960; Clark, 1965; Hinshelwood & Manning, 1979), need necessarily apply. They may well do so, but if so, a reason must be given as to why they are appropriate in a particular setting and suited to the social and emotional needs of this particular clientele (Johnson, 1981).

There is, for example, no prior assumption of a need for 'therapy', and the language of personal change can be quite informal, ordinary and non-technical. Nor is an explicit community focus necessarily central; for those who wish to live down their past, or simply to move on to better things, an expectation of community commitment and participation may even be counter-productive.

The concept of a PIE could then equally apply to those environments that are created with an awareness of particular psychological deficits, and planned and managed to minimise difficult or problematic behaviour, and contain any risks. Examples of this kind of environment might include some specialist residential communities for individuals with very specific physical or learning difficulties. These environments can be both planned and enabling, even where there is no actual change intended in the particular underlying area of difficulty that characterises the service users or members of the community. They simply aim to allow the individuals concerned to get on with other areas of their lives, no longer held back by infringements upon their autonomy or dignity or the disruption and conflicts that their disability or disempowerment otherwise entails. They are, to that extent 'prosthetic environments'.

In the paper that originally proposed the term PIE (Johnson & Haigh, 2010), it was therefore argued that there is as yet no single or particular school of thought or of human understanding that necessarily underpins or informs a PIE. There is no one set of beliefs that the staff of a PIE need to sign up to, and no overall view of the nature of human nature. It might, therefore:

'*... be any form of psychological theory that might inform the work of the staff, from psychodynamics to behaviourism, from Gestalt to evolutionary psychology, Transactional Analysis, Dialectical Behavioural Therapy, Neuro-Linguistic Programming to existential humanism, and all points between* *and beyond. It is perhaps arguable that a meditation space or retreat founded on the more psychologically oriented faiths, such as Buddhism, might qualify.'* (Johnson & Haigh, 2010)

One thing, however, that we can say with confidence is that, whether in a prison, a night shelter, or even an acute ward, or wherever safety and management of risk is a key concern, a genuinely constructive environment always aims to do more than simply contain challenging behaviour. A PIE or PIPE will aim to use the potential for change that resides in all human beings for the pursuit of some wider or future goal, whether it be the reduction of re-offending, a positive attitude to learning, developing better interpersonal relationships, or engagement with formal treatment and therapy.

The PIE approach can therefore perhaps best be thought of not as a new model in itself, but rather as a tool or framework to encourage creative and responsive thinking on the part of the staff team. While it is important to stress the role of the staff team in thinking afresh about the needs of the client group, this not to say that service users, carers, volunteers and graduates will not be involved in such reflection, only that there is no prescribed way, such as the 'community meeting' in a TC, by which that should happen.

Further questions

There are two further questions that need answering.

First: is being psychologically informed in itself enough to guarantee more humane treatment? As one cautious critic has suggested, brainwashing is thoroughly psychologically informed. If that may seem an absurd extreme, it may well be, nevertheless, that in addition to psychological insights we need to include some form of value statement. In homelessness services, such values are already embedded in the service model by the Quality Assurance Framework for Supporting People funding (House of Commons, 2010). Is there a need for something comparable in other areas where PIEs or PIPEs might go?

The second question is this: are there limits to the applicability of the PIE concept? Where the post-war concept of a TC was unable to go, the more flexible and adaptable concept of a PIE may now be applied. With its stress on reflective practice in frontline services, the PIE approach – along with its counterpart the PIPE, for high risk or secure settings – aims to revitalise discussion over how best to manage the psychological and emotional needs of some of those most excluded from the mainstream of society, and to support them into recovery. However, one key aspect of a PIE, and an essential requirement for a PIPE, is that there should be a coherent, defined environment that is managed and so can be planned in order for that planning to be more 'psychologically' informed.

What are we then to say of those many social environments where the members of the community themselves have the largest say in how they run their own lives, not as planned by any other group, but self-directing, as individuals living their own lives? Or of all those environments where people come together and are organised, but for a different primary purpose, be it education or leisure, work or worship? This, after all, is the community at large, where most of us live most of our lives.

However, with increasing recognition of the wider social determinants of health, mental health and well-being (Marmot & Wilkinson, 2003; Department of Health, 2009a; Milton, 2010), it becomes both necessary and possible to explore a wider range of issues that impact upon individual and community well-being. To address the wider social determinants of public health, mental health and well-being, we will need new concepts that can recognise and promote positive social relationships and social capital on a broader canvas.

Here we must go beyond the notion of a planned environment, and we will need to introduce a second, and considerably broader concept – the 'enabling environment'.

What do we mean by 'psychology'?

It is important to establish exactly what we mean by the word 'psychology' when discussing PIEs. To over-simplify for a moment, we might suggest that there are two potentially divergent meanings of psychology. The question is not which is correct, but how to harness them both most constructively.

On the one hand, psychology is shorthand for 'psychological science' – a branch of science characterised by the application of proper scientific methods of enquiry to the mind, behaviour, reactions and human relationships. The common thread in 'psychological science' is an allegiance to a broad notion of science as rigorous, universalist and methodologically sound.

In the context of working with vulnerable people, or those in need of help, one of the great strengths of psychodynamic thinking is that it takes very seriously the idea that there are emotional defences – the 'resistance' – against the upset provoked by growing psychological awareness, and tries to work on those issues first. By contrast, one of the great strengths of more positivist or behaviourist psychology is that it has no truck with resistance, but simply asserts what is well evidenced, and teaches that.

Humanistic psychology is sometimes described as 'the third force' in psychology, coming as it did after the establishment of psychoanalytic and behavioural approaches. Humanistic psychology is not a specific technique or school, but rather a perspective in psychology that focuses on and sets most store by the aspects of our existence that are uniquely human, such as potential, meaning, value, personal responsibility, choice, individuality and self-expression. More humanistic approaches in therapy or treatment tend to work to support and endorse these features and capacities in the lives of those coming for assistance.

Work to engage marginalised and excluded individuals, those with entrenched difficulties, and/or those who are especially wary of authority or care services, may often need to start with such issues, to achieve the engagement with support that may even need to precede the offer of shelter. This may, for example, mean that the therapist gives at least equal weight to the person's strength and goals – their assets. Humanistic psychology, like behaviourism, tends to keep at arm's length the medical model of psychiatry, and typically aims for a less pathology-focused view of the person.

A key ingredient in this approach is the encounter between therapist and client and the possibilities for dialogue. Humanistic psychology practitioners tend, therefore, to allow their own personalities and concerns to become part of the engagement process, rather than attempting to remain neutral as simply technique providers, as behaviourist approaches imply, or to become a blank screen on which clients may project their own concerns, as psychoanalytic theory typically proposes.

In some respects, therefore, humanistic approaches offer an alternative, but humanistic practitioners are typically holistic, and aim to integrate a wide (or 'eclectic') range of insights and specific techniques, as appropriate to each individual's needs and circumstances. It may be just as accurate and helpful to see humanistic approaches, not as a distinct third force, but rather as the fertile meeting ground between the other two. In fact, of course, all these different schools and approaches draw from each other hugely, and more skilled and confident practitioners may draw on techniques and insights that underlie them all. However, crucially, all schools recognise that learning and unlearning are both most effectively achieved in some kind of helpful relationship, and especially in a group.

Ordinary psychology and human empathy

That, then, is one meaning of psychology, but there is another. Psychology can also be conceived more naturalistically, as the attempt to understand our own and other people's minds, and their reactions to events; to look for the personal meaning in another's behaviour (or our own). We are born, it seems, with a capacity for empathy that is intrinsic and fundamental to the nature of being human. Although there are some in whom this capacity is lacking or damaged, or who have had the capacity drummed out of them, we see this as a pathology, a malformation, something to be explained and treated with special care.

When we are calling for a more 'mindful' or 'psychologically informed' environment in those services that are by their nature working with individuals who have suffered some degree of trauma in their lives, we are not necessarily calling, therefore, for exceptional skills or knowledge or effort, but only for the restitution and recognition of ordinary human responsiveness. Some things in life require highly specialist knowledge and skills, and qualifications – such as being a doctor or a CORGI-approved gas engineer. Human responsiveness, fortunately, is not one of them.

Psychology in this sense (the ability of humans and some other higher primates to make sense of each other's actions, take them into account and work with them for co-operation or conflict) has evident evolutionary survival advantages.

Such everyday or 'folk' psychology may be deliberate and conscious, explicit, thoughtful and reflective, but much of it is intuitive and 'pre-conscious', ie. it is something that we have never consciously thought about (Pinker, 1997; Gladwell, 2005; Marcus, 2008; Kahnemann, 2011). Hence the scope for psychoanalysts and anthropologists to hypothesise some form of individual and/or collective 'unconscious', and for social theorists to suggest that much of this pre-conscious intuition is learned and/or socially constructed (Berger

& Luckmann, 1966; Carroll, 2000; Cromby, 2005). Whatever the merits of and evidence for particular theories, it seems undeniable that much of human emotion, behaviour and cognition is grounded in these foundations, which are pre-theoretical, even pre-conscious – although, to some degree at least, open to conscious exploration.

Yet psychology in this broader sense – or 'mind-mindedness', as it has also been called – can be encouraged or discouraged, valued or dismissed, used or sidelined. Psychology can even be deliberately expelled from an area of academic study – and only rehabilitated when the model that has rejected it is questioned and loses its dominance.

Both of these conceptions of psychology seem to be equally useful, and each has its place. Academic, laboratory research and clinical psychology and psychotherapy clearly have a great deal to contribute to enriching human understanding, but it is perhaps only when they work together that we will find a thoroughly psychologically informed environment.

Editor's comment:
A wider approach

These chapters have presented an overview of the nature of trauma and its impact on our lives, the nature of recovery, and the crucial role of community and the wider social environment. We have offered an account of the complexity of traumatising experiences, and especially of what we term complex traumas, where any original overwhelming stress has been compounded by repeated life experience of conflict, distrust and alienation, until the defensive patterns of response eventually become embedded and self-fulfilling, and increasingly hard to interrupt. Yet we have also seen how interactions with others subsequently can help or hinder recovery, and the importance of the psycho-social environment to rebuilding a sense of belonging.

Nevertheless, if recovery from even the extreme versions of traumatised experience lies in reintegration into a community, then the nature and quality of the social environments of contemporary society must also have some bearing on the capacity for recovery and reintegration.

Up to this point, we have focused principally on the efforts of specialist services and approaches. Here, we have argued, we can see emerging various recurring themes, and we have suggested that the consistency with which these themes interweave throughout the narrative may in itself be telling us something valuable about the nature of the problems being addressed.

We suggest, in other words, that the evolution of sensitive and constructive responses to a problem sheds some light on the underlying nature of the problem, which complements what might be gleaned from clinical trials and laboratory studies. These stories provide food for thought for those wanting to grasp the nature of the problem, and especially of course for those wishing to draw inspiration for their own efforts to tackle such problems in their own work.

Nevertheless, are there perhaps still deeper underlying issues and themes? In particular, if it is the case – as we suggest – that trauma lies on a continuum with ordinary, everyday stress, which affects us all, then we might well want to ask if there are some aspects of the recovery environment that are relevant to us all. Are there then some underlying principles in what constitutes or what creates a more healthy social environment, based more upon the importance of relatedness or 'social capital' and the encouragement of emotional intelligence?

The final chapter of this book describes the attempts being made under the auspices of the Royal College of Psychiatrists to identify just such principles and to refine and develop an awareness of them as a touchstone measure – even a quality standard – for constructive communities. This initiative, which goes by the name of 'enabling environments', looks for the underlying dynamics of relatedness and belonging not in techniques or even in social skills, but in the underlying values that bind together a community, whether in a hospital ward or care home, or in a church community, a workplace, or on a housing estate.

The humanistic approach in psychology has helped to re-focus our attention on those aspects of our lives that are uniquely human, such as potential, meaning, achievements and values, and we have repeatedly seen evidence for the importance of working with people's aspirations and self-esteem. Our final perspective, then, is that of society's values, and the extent to which a clearer focus on such values can help to foster enabling environments across the whole spectrum of experience, from those most troubled and marginalised, to the rest of us – the community at large.

Chapter 23

Enabling environments, public health and human values

Robin Johnson and Rex Haigh[1]

'The welfare state that was built up after the great economic crises of the 1930s was designed to address Britain's material needs – for jobs, homes, healthcare and pensions. It was assumed that people's emotional needs would be met by close knit families and communities. Sixty years later, psychological needs have become as pressing as material ones: the risk of loneliness and isolation; the risk of mental illness; the risk of being left behind. New solutions are needed … to equip people with the resilience they'll need to get by in uncertain times.' (Young Foundations, 2009)

Community mental health

What exactly do we mean by community mental health?

Is it essentially the post-war programme of hospital closures and 'care in the community' (Griffiths, 1988)? Is it simply standard mental healthcare – medication, counselling etc – but now delivered through domiciliary visits to the patient's own home, or in clinics or care homes, instead of in hospitals?

Is it more a matter of specialist mental health services engaging more fully with other community agencies to maintain vulnerable individuals in an ordinary life, a home and a job? Is it about encouraging inter-agency

1 The following article has been adapted from material first published in a trilogy of papers titled 'Social psychiatry and social policy for the 21st century', in *Mental Health and Social Inclusion* **14** (4) 30–35; **15** (1) 17–23; **15** (2) 57–65.

partnership work with housing, leisure services, faith communities, and the wide variety of institutions and agencies that make up 'the community'? Is this about joined-up government, a continuation of the social exclusion approach, pooled 'community budgets' and a string of other initiatives aimed at getting frontline services to work together (Social Exclusion Unit, 2004; Department of Health, 2009a; Department for Communities and Local Government/National Mental Health Development Unit, 2010)?

Or is it something more radical still, and concerned with the mental health of the community as a whole; an aspect of public health intended to encourage a more enlightened, less stressed and self-destructive society? Is it a response to the more pervasive malaise that the Young Foundations report (2009) quotation above identifies? Is this the so-called happiness agenda? Is this perhaps an aspect of the elusive 'Big Society' (Norman, 2010) that the current UK government and some in the opposition (Milliband, 2011; Hansard, 2011) have said they wish to see?

Or if it perhaps needs to be all of the above blended together, how do they all fit together? How in practice might we find or create a single framework to unite or bridge them all?

We have suggested that the impact of poor mental health, from stress to trauma to psychiatric disorder, may be far more pervasive throughout society than depression and anxiety, and the remedy may be both far deeper and far wider. Where then is the 'big idea', the practical, integrating agenda for positive community mental health for the 21st century?

The development of the enabling environment approach

In Chapter 21, we described the renewed ambition to develop a new kind of community mental health, or a more social psychiatry. Building upon the development since the Second World War of the therapeutic community (TC) as an approach, the demands of a changing world now mean that we must look for similarly humane principles to realise a vision for community mental health that takes into its scope the needs of the wider community and the population at large.

Since 2002, the Community of Communities' quality network has been developed by the Royal College of Psychiatrists (RCP). Its original aim was to identify an agreed set of standards by which TCs operate – a professionally agreed specification of what constitutes TC practice (RCP, 2010). This was to provide consistency, especially for research purposes and future commissioning, and it could be further developed as a basis for a future regulatory framework.

Since 2005, the Community of Communities project went from specifying operational standards to identifying the values that underlie the attitudes and understandings of those working in the field. These values and standards are specific to those communities that wish to follow the TC principles. As a result, we now have a set of TC 'core standards' for member communities, which explicitly reference and reflect the core values associated with them.

However, there are potentially very many other forms of community and socially minded enterprise that are striving in their own way to create the kind of emotional and social environment that is most conducive to their particular goals and aspirations. The role of shared values is clearly not restricted to the small cluster of explicit communities that identify as TCs, and it is important not to exclude those other constructive communities and approaches that do not, or would not, see themselves as TCs, or to imply that only TCs could make a valuable contribution to the lives of their members.

The Community of Communities project therefore agreed to the formation of a further working group, whose task was to identify comparable core principles and standards that would be applicable in non-TC settings. These principles needed to embrace a broader range of concepts – concepts within which communities that identified themselves as TCs could recognise themselves, but so too could many others besides.

It was clearly not appropriate to simply take the axioms of the TC movement and apply them to a wider range of settings, even in a watered down form. Instead, the group had to start afresh, with discussions of first principles, based partly on practitioner's knowledge of 'what works', partly on the growing body of research evidence that now underpins our understanding of what works, and partly on exploration of the standards set by other regulatory frameworks.

Enabling environments (EEs) became the name of the project, and the Enabling Environment Development Group (EEDG) became the name of the working group.

Deliberately holding in mind a very wide set of possible settings, from wards to workplaces, schools, housing projects, prisons and places of faith, the EEDG working party set about defining what seemed to be the core issues or features of a constructive or 'enabling' environment.

It was equally clear that the defining characteristics of an EE approach could not be based on any particular psychological theory, or on the deliberations of a staff team, but rather on the common threads which, in the eyes of ordinary people, bind communities together. These, it was felt, could be divided into task-based and values-based themes. Task-based issues were dependent on the particular activity or sector; only the underlying values ran through all sectors.

A values-based approach

This, of course, is clearly not merely ambitious, but also contentious. Can it really be possible, in a pluralist world, let alone one in which conflict as much as consensus drives social change, both to identify a single set of values that express the wish for community, and also have the relative objectivity that we normally expect of healthcare terminology? Are not all values relative, too unreliable to form a basis for healthcare innovations? Is this ambition not philosophically flawed, and therefore doomed to failure? Three things, however, suggest otherwise.

First, there is increasing recognition that health, under the guise of a degree of consensus so broad that it is not even seen as consensus, is an endeavour imbued with values. The rapidly growing new profession of medical ethics is testament to the need to reveal and debate the underlying ethical premises on which medical judgments are made. Psychiatry in particular has to be clear about its judgments of value (Widdershoven *et al*, 2008; Fulford, 2010), and since, as we know, there is no health without mental health (RCP, 2010), there is therefore some basis for considering all healthcare values as shared values (Fleck, 1979). There may not be after all any fundamental difference between health values and social values. At least there seems to be a basis for re-examining the social determinants, impacts and contexts of mental health as a whole, and in the explicitly value-laden language of priorities, costs and benefits.

Second, there is growing evidence that we can substantiate some values statements with evidence. We have plentiful science now to confirm the impact of distress and social factors such as isolation, relationship stress and exclusion on health through an impaired immune system reaction, leading to slower healing of physical wounds. Through carefully designed experiments, we can now simulate experiences of rejection and exclusion in laboratory conditions, which can be traced and measured even at a neuro-anatomical level, and we find that it is the pain centres of the brain that are activated. We also have carefully evaluated social policy programmes for initiatives and pilots that demonstrate, for example, that choice and empowerment, whether at individual or whole community level, improve satisfaction and well-being. These may be values statements, but to coin a phrase, we hold these emotional truths to be well evidenced.

Finally, as we shift our focus from healthcare alone to the wider range of social policy and community cohesion, we do find, in the social policy frameworks that govern our practice, a relatively consistent cluster of values underpinning what we seem to want from our lives in the community. Certainly in social values there are inconsistencies verging on paradox or outright contradiction. But there is sufficient of a common core here for us to tease these common core social values out, explore and even propose them as a framework that seems on the whole to reflect what it is that we look for in a healthy workplace, a welcoming community, a caring hospital.

This is essentially an empirical question – to what extent can we discern common values in the public evaluation of, and in the operating principles of, the regulatory bodies that govern the key services that impact on social welfare and the common good? If we can do so, the more metaphysical questions over where these values come from – whether they are sanctioned by a deity, immanent in our evolved social natures, necessarily implied by the very concept of 'morality', or represent some form of collective existential choice – may be addressed elsewhere.

For present purposes, they would provide a basic foundation for a practical programme to explore how the role of the social environment may lie at the heart of psychological well-being, and so to locate mental health at the heart of social policy. There is and probably can never be a single uncontested concept of community and common purpose in how people may live, work and be together in the social world (MacIntyre, 1985; Hoggett, 2009). But from a reading of the 'grey literature' of policy statements from government departments and statutory regulatory bodies, cutting across or running through the different 'jurisdictions' of a wide range of sectors, certain themes, principles or standards seem to consistently underlie and articulate what were seen to be the main issues in positive practice.

The EE's core elements

The EEDG working party concluded that it was possible to identify 10 broad clusters of concerns and aspirations. For example, we might suggest that, as a general rule, a positively enabling environment would be one:

- in which the nature and the quality of relationships between participants or members would be recognised and highly valued
- where the participants share some measure of responsibility for the environment as a whole, and especially for their own part in it
- where all participants – staff, volunteers and service users alike – are equally valued and supported in their particular contribution
- where engagement and purposeful activity is encouraged
- where there are opportunities for creativity and initiative, whether spontaneous or planned
- where decision-making is transparent, and both formal and informal leadership roles are acknowledged
- where power or authority is clearly accountable and open to discussion
- where any formal rules or informal expectations of behaviour are clear, or if unclear, there is good reason for it
- where behaviour, even when potentially disruptive, is seen as meaningful, as a communication to be understood.

What is more, within each specific area of human social activity, there now appears to be considerable direct and/or corroborating evidence for the validity and efficacy of these underlying principles.

From common values to shared standards

When identifying truly enabling environments, exactly 'what works' will clearly have to be broad, consistent, and yet adaptable. However, this is not simply because there might be a range of possibly conflicting values to be encompassed: this is not solely a matter of a compromise between universalist principles and a necessarily messy pluralism in practice.

It is also important in principle that the members, stakeholders, staff and users of any service in any setting should identify what they want and what they find in their particular environment. Within any set of broad concerns and aspirations, it is still necessary for the participants in each setting to take 'ownership' and specify and translate these concerns in a way that is suitable and most meaningful for them.

What the EE approach offers, in proposing a set of specified themes and standards, is a vocabulary and tool that individuals, groups and communities can use to articulate their own aspirations for a more constructive EE. However, it is essential that, within each community or setting, the participants should be able to agree between them the kind of environment that they want, and the adoption of any local set of standards by any group or community needs to be a voluntary action. To that extent, therefore, the stress on shared reflection from the psychologically informed environment (PIE) approach appears to be just as valid here – though the nature and format of that reflectiveness needs to vary, according to the opportunities in the situation. The extent to which, and even the means by which, the ground rules of participation and belonging are open to discussion and renegotiation will vary between primary schools, homelessness hostels and hospital wards.

For example, there is clearly a debate to be had about how far any care environment (such as a hospital ward or a residential care home) should be protective and controlling, or how far it needs to be permissive and supportive of risk-taking and experimentation. The core concern is therefore about a balance of risk, but the appropriate balance will vary according to the setting. For example, the balance of acceptable risk and individual initiative will be very different in a prison setting to that of a housing estate, or an old people's home. It must be open to the members of each community or group to agree how much challenge and protection is right for them. To some extent, in fact, it may be the act of discussion and consensus-building that is the essential step in the process.

As a rule, EEs do not go out of their way to create conditions of adversity for their members. However, there can be individuals and groups within any one environment who thrive on adversity. Indeed, many would say that a certain amount of challenge builds character and resilience. In a learning environment such as a school, therefore, or perhaps a psychotherapeutic treatment centre, experiences of tackling challenges may be essential, and removing them would be counter-productive. In a still less formal environment such as a housing estate, individuals will want the right to make their own decisions over their lives, and secure containment need consist only of some shared understanding over how far one individual's enjoyment may be allowed to intrude on others' rights to their own. What constitutes unacceptable, excessive, intrusive or antisocial behaviour must be defined by the community itself.

EEs in practice

Having established the core principles of the EE approach, the EEDG group then undertook a preliminary consultation exercise to assess the likely interest in the initiative, and it was clear from the responses that it was broadly welcomed (Northern Housing Consortium, 2009). A number of services indicated a willingness to pilot the accreditation procedure. The majority of these 'early adopters' were care services operating in specialist areas, principally in mental health, rather than the broader range of community services or agencies.

Early results nevertheless indicated that these 'early adopter' agencies found the process of measuring themselves against these standards to be quite useful in itself. Initial feedback from the pilots was again very positive; staff and service users alike reported with some enthusiasm that the process of assessing their service by these criteria was itself a positive experience. In particular, the expectation that service users should also give their views has opened up a discussion that is constructive in its own right. It seems the process of assessment, where it creates dialogue, is itself a process of change.

The practical applications of EE standards

There are several possible ways to use the EE standards and operational criteria in practice. In many situations, a simple awareness of best practice and a shared language to articulate an ambition to operate more constructively may be all that is achievable. Here, the EE vocabulary of shared values offers a common language to aid communications and mutual understanding within and between services, agencies and communities.

In other instances, however, services, institutions or communities might choose to assess themselves consciously and deliberately against these criteria. Services could then declare and register this explicit ambition with the RCP as 'aspiring EEs', and then work towards their agreed goals in their own way. The RCP's EEs project support team, once fully operational, could also provide or suggest support and training through accredited affiliates. The EEDG would therefore develop a 'portfolio' for self-assessment and improvement to be used by services in specific sectors. There would also be the option of peer review with service users and staff, using the same portfolio approach for evidence.

Where appropriate, adoption of the EE approach and the portfolio of evidence might then be recognised and allowed as part of the more formal external quality assurance assessments of other regulatory bodies. With national regulatory bodies moving generally towards lighter-touch and risk-based assessments (Better Regulation Executive, 2009), a declared ambition to achieve especially high standards might appeal to many services wishing to commit to a stronger sense of community spirit and public health, and to reference such ambitions in future discussions with commissioners, professionals and service users.

However, for agencies that wish to pursue and demonstrate service improvement by a still more rigorous and objective assessment, the project would also develop its own formal assessment process, leading then to a formal accreditation and an award of 'EE status'. Assessment would be based on a portfolio of evidence, but with on-site visits from trained assessors and discussions with staff, service users and stakeholders, for external verification. The RCP is willing to remain the formal accrediting body – but equally willing to relinquish or share that role with any other suitable agency.

EEs, public health and the intermediary role of institutions

The public health programme of the coalition government so far has two principle focuses.

First, there is the stated intention (Department of Health, 2010) to give a lead role and a significant slice of the healthcare budget to local authorities, to integrate public health initiatives at local level with their wider role in analysing the needs of the local population and commissioning services (Lyons, 2006). This approach builds upon a steady stream of policy pronouncements over many years (Social Exclusion Unit 2004; Association of Directors of Adult Services, 2008; HM Treasury, 2010) that have stressed the need for agencies to work together, to consider shared outcomes and partnerships in delivery – especially to meet more complex needs.

Second, less attention has so far been given to what is promised to be a series of 'responsibility deals' (Lansley, 2009; Department of Health, 2011a) with industry, aiming to develop a partnership between government and business that balances regulation with responsible action, to address public health problems such as poor diet, alcohol abuse and lack of exercise. This second approach builds upon attempts to promote the corporate social responsibility of business, industry and commerce. In a climate where any commercial enterprise can find itself suddenly at the mercy of a firestorm of bad publicity over the social consequences of apparent 'efficiency' – outsourcing and child labour, for example – responsibility deals agreed with government offer some degree of protection (Kytle, 2005).

Taken together, however, this two-pronged approach begins to resemble in some respects the earlier work of the former social inclusion programmes – that is, each seeks changes in the way society's institutions themselves work, rather than relying solely on tardy and costly remedial action for those who have succumbed or 'fallen through the net'.

Responsibility deals and public health programmes similarly address the health and/or vulnerability of the population as a whole, and, whether at national or at local level, they seek to ensure that all agencies play their part in maintaining the health of the nation. Whereas social exclusion policy was focused on integrating the marginalised, both public health and now the EE approach are equally concerned for the healthier integration of the majority.

The EE approach, which deliberately sets out to bridge the values statements of different sectors and the jurisdictions of different regulatory bodies, aims to provide a common language for partnerships, and for a new generation of responsibility deals at local level.

Community and the social determinants of health

The decline of traditional community and the weakening of 'social capital' is widely seen as part of the general malaise that accentuates individual mental health problems. We also know that group and neighbourhood effects can be as powerful as individual characteristics in the incubation of antisocial and/or other self-harming behaviour (Lewin, 1948), and that neighbourhood-level interventions are as effective as individual-focused ones (Griggs *et al*, 2008).

In the last few years, the Department for Communities and Local Government (CLG) has produced several good practice guidance documents on community development, intended for local community development workers. Perhaps most interesting of all – and of obvious relevance to community mental health work, from public mental well-being to secondary care – was a fascinating guidance document (CLG, 2009) on how to recognise and promote 'meaningful interaction' at face-to-face, citizen to citizen level. This guidance – intended to combat the potential for extremism within marginalised communities – suggests that there are four levels of interaction that are valuable, which they characterise as grounding interactions, 'banal' (sic) interactions, opportunity interactions, and growth interactions.

'Grounding interactions are about consolidating one's [own] identity and values, take place with people with whom one shares a history, and help to build individual self-confidence and pride.'

Banal interactions *'are about consolidating one's external environment, and take place with people with whom one shares a community. [They] are typically fairly superficial – saying hello in the street or exchanging chit-chat. They help develop a sense of belonging and contribute to good community relations'.*

'Opportunity interactions are about broadening one's external environment, and take place with people with whom one shares potential benefits. Networks, self-help groups, campaigns and committees can bring people from different backgrounds together and open up new opportunities.'

'Growth interactions are about broadening one's identity and values, and take place with people with whom one shares curiosity. It is through growth interactions that people change the way they see themselves and others, and find new things in common.' (CLG, 2009b)

This was seen as a community cohesion issue – it was in fact based on earlier work by the Commission for Racial Equality – and so was largely ignored by mental health services or other welfare agencies concerned with inclusion practice. This unfortunate silo-ing of our imaginations illustrates nicely the need for something like Big Society thinking, as a programme to bring together broader thinking on where we really want to be as a society. A sense of belonging (CLG, 2009), and a hunger for more meaningful interactions, is not just an issue for minority communities. Many members of the indigenous community need that too.

Communities and their social lives

Where agencies, services and networks in communities wish to become more cohesively focused on the social dimensions of health and well-being, the EE vocabulary offers a latter-day Rosetta Stone that provides a common language of concerns, not just for 'recipients' of specific services but, equally necessary, between other 'providers' to bridge the concerns of divergent agencies. The EE approach consciously aims to span 'natural' or informal communities, and the institutions, agencies and services that are found there. We believe that it may even develop as a mechanism for reconciling the individualistic and the communitarian strands of Big Society practice (Norman, 2010) with the broader programme of public health and social inclusion practice, at institutional levels.

Whereas 'the national health' is something that we pay for in our taxes, 'relational health' (Jordan, 2001; Frey *et al*, 2005) is something we do for ourselves – but also, can only do with other people; relational health is intrinsically reciprocal – even when one party to the interaction may struggle to reciprocate (CLG/NMHDU, 2010). However, this does not mean that relational health is essentially individual. It is a many-layered co-production, and the agencies and social groups, the intermediary structures within and through which we live, may help or hinder. The agencies, social structures, organisational cultures and media stereotypes currently infusing our social world play a huge role in fostering or compromising such relations. The EE approach, focused as it is on the social and collective aspects, aims for collective expressions of the aspiration for more connectedness.

If there is ever to be such a things as a 'Big Society', then it will need a practical programme, over and beyond a general feeling of solidarity in tough times, and a preference for volunteering and for delivery of services by the voluntary sector and not-for-profit groups.

The question is not so much whether we are looking for a Big Society, to make up for welfare cuts, but whether we perhaps need a 'Still Bigger Society' to make good the deficits that the Young Foundations and World Health Organization reports are describing.

We have seen the erosion of community, the hollowing out of working relationships into codified and instrumental units of efficiency, and the increasing mechanisation of care so that it is now conceived not as fellow feeling, but as a thing to be delivered, like pizza. We now need a reconstructive framework that puts relationships and connectedness at the heart of all future progress. It is the ambition of the EE project to offer a voice and a vocabulary for the effort to create a more richly textured, deeper society.

Future prospects and wider relevance

The EE approach is as broad as it is ambitious. There seems little doubt that it will evolve, perhaps radically, as we draw other sectors and agencies into the task of identifying common ground underlying so many different perspectives and jurisdictions. Yet what is most ambitious here is not the attempt to bridge and integrate medico-technical and social values systems but the attempt to find core statements of purpose that are 'cross platform' – that can be applied across a wide variety of settings, each of which typically comes under the jurisdiction of other bodies whose concerns may dovetail, but whose technical language rarely does.

Summary: connecting threads

As the 21st century progresses we face new challenges in the development of a social psychiatry that is suited to its times. We are increasingly aware of the social determinants of poor health, the positive role of social capital, and the negative impact of social exclusion. Moreover, there is a growing sense that mental health underlies many of the remaining physical health problems of our age – that there is no health without mental health – and, for example, many 'medically unexplained symptoms' are likely to be best addressed through psychosocial means. Earlier clear-cut distinctions between medical interventions and socio-economic goals now seem less tenable.

We have set out to trace these historical developments and how they are interwoven with broader social policy in order to put in context and outline three emerging concepts (namely, PIEs, psychologically informed planned environments and EEs) that are attempting to recognise the 'micro-social' dimensions of health. This all indicates an agenda for a new social psychiatry, which, however, needs new tools to face these new challenges. This chapter has attempted to suggest that community mental health and a new social psychiatry must be consciously positioned at the heart of all efforts to promote public health, reduce social exclusion, create sustainable communities, and develop a vibrant economy for the future.

Where the concept of a TC seemed unable to go, the concept of a PIE can now be more flexibly applied. However, to address the broader social determinants of health, mental health and well-being, we also need concepts that can recognise and promote positive social relationships and social capital more broadly. Here, the concept of an EE attempts to transcend the distinction between treatment agencies and the wider world. These EE standards and setting-specific criteria will inevitably be modified with further feedback as other sectors are drawn into the fold. Indeed, they will need to be kept under review and will evolve as new 'members' contribute to the process. This is, and will remain, 'a work in progress'.

There is much work still to be done to develop perhaps a whole range of PIEs, and to provide a range of different working models that communities can adopt, to agree and guide their aspirations for a more human-centred world. The search for a new social psychiatry has barely begun.

Chapter 24
Conclusion

Robin Johnson

Homo sum; humani nil a me alienum puto

I am a human being; I see nothing human as foreign to me

A recent exchange from a Radio 4 broadcast on the Today programme's news slot (BBC, 2009) may serve to illustrate the issues lying at the heart of this book.

The neuroscientist Steven Rose was invited to the studio and asked to comment on a newly published study of nine mentally disordered offenders that had suggested, based on the results of brain scans, that 'psychopaths' brains are physically different from ours. The researchers *'claimed that these findings were compelling evidence for the biological basis of criminal psychopathy'*.

Professor Rose gently pointed out that what all these individuals actually had in common was a long history of incarceration, substance abuse, and probably of treatment with highly invasive psychiatric medication. If their brains now look different on a scan, what then was cause, and what effect?

This exchange reveals two broad beliefs now so commonplace that they barely seemed to need questioning: that psychopaths are biologically different from the rest of us, and that it is their (and our) brains that explain how they (and we) behave.

These two popular myths and misconceptions – fuelled not just by the media, but by the well-meaning research community and even many in the medical profession – go to the heart of the thinking that this book has tried to challenge. In these pages, we have tried to demonstrate that even such extremes of human behaviour as outright psychopathy nevertheless lie at one end of a wide spectrum of traumatised lives, and at the other end of the same spectrum, in a milder form, are disturbances that underlie many of the social problems that bedevil modern society and are responsible for those who 'fail to thrive'.

Trauma and cycles

The central subject of this book is trauma, and our ambition has been to introduce a broad range of new perspectives that can help us understand and trace the conditions that can create, and the conditions that can heal, psychological and emotional trauma.

A key realisation has been that psychological trauma is not something that rapidly becomes an event in the past. On the contrary, it is the constant replaying and re-enactment of traumatised scenarios that may be the principal psychological consequence of trauma. These may reach their peak, and are seen at their most extreme, in the dysfunctional and disabling behaviours of those who might be diagnosed with personality disorder, chronic post-traumatic stress, or, as we prefer, complex trauma, and the history of unsatisfying and impoverished relationships that these people often experience.

If trauma interrupts otherwise healthy human development, the response to trauma can still be seen as a natural process, and part of the wide repertoire with which nature has equipped us to prepare us for hostile conditions, even from birth or pre-birth. The nature of trauma is therefore central to human development, a result of the brain's natural plasticity responding to events, and to one extent or another it plays a part in the development of us all. A growing appreciation of this phenomena is part of the new understanding of the nature of humanity via the emerging biological model of epigenetics.

The cyclical, self-reinforcing nature of these experiences, conscious or unconscious, can now be understood and recognised both at a neurological level – in the habituated pathways of dense neural connectivity that intense experience creates – and in the unwanted repetitive patterns of behaviour, emotion and thought that may then run through all our subsequent relationships and social lives.

However, at any stage – and this is crucial – there may be some event or series of events that intervenes, that breaks the cycle, and that changes the course of events. The predictability of the course of events that leads, apparently remorselessly, from trauma to disorder is more a product of our way of pigeon-holing problems, our approach to gathering data and research, than it is of inevitable consequences. Instead, we can now see that what we do over these intervening years matters; it changes things.

The effects of trauma can also be seen in the everyday social lives which we humans have developed around us. We may be fundamentally social creatures, but we are only slowly unlearning the social and cultural imprinting that our species owes to an early time in our history, when our lives were often more brutal, and our social lives more tribal. One aspect of that is that we have very varying degrees of tolerance for the individuals around us who may be challenging and demanding.

Yet the range of social environments in contemporary society includes a complex matrix of organisations and agencies whose whole role and purpose is to help, nurture and guide towards success the infant, child, student, colleague, client, neighbour, patient, or whatever role we may play at any point in time, in any context.

The extent to which those various agencies are able to recognise, understand and work with the problematic and conflicted behaviour that some will show can make all the difference to those individuals' capacity for growth and learning, taking up the new opportunities offered, moving up and out into emotional and social recovery and fully rounded lives. Those who fail to thrive are as much failed by society as they are by early nurture and neurological development.

One essential argument of this book begins with the realisation that our behaviour, even our most problematic behaviour, cannot be determined by our genes to any meaningful degree. Instead, our main or typical behaviour patterns – our personalities – develop throughout childhood in a complex interaction with our emotional and social environment, in which both neural connectivity and biochemistry play their part actively – made possible by our genetic endowment, but not predetermined by it.

The new emerging understanding of human development, which is the principal focus of Section one has, we argue, finally resolved not only the old divide between mind and body, but also the old distinctions between nature and nurture. We can now see more clearly the pervasive influence of social processes alongside and in equal measure with the biological, in the creation of human nature.

This now focuses our attentions not only on early years – admittedly our most formative years, and those when we are most vulnerable to the impact of traumatising experience – but throughout all the years of development, and beyond into adult life. We are constantly changing; not merely in our thoughts and our relationships with others in the social world, but also at a biological and neurological level.

Section two is full of examples of social action – or social practice – by which means thoughtful and engaged individuals have been finding new ways to assist those who are struggling with the burden or the risk of trauma and psychiatric disorder.

These examples of civil society at work are the equivalent of the laboratory and ethological studies of animals. We argue that they are as legitimate a contribution to the scientific understanding of human nature as any studies from the laboratory or the field trip, and they can show us aspects of human potential to which animal studies, however insightful on our biological nature, cannot do justice. We can certainly accept that humans are animals, but we must also accept that, as animals, we are quite unusual.

Where Section one considered the theory, and Section two the practice, Section three then looked towards the future.

The future

We can look forward to exciting and thought-provoking new discoveries in neuroscience, which will help us understand better the frailties to which we as a species are prone, and the constructive interventions that may result from a better understanding. However, it is beyond the scope of a book such as this to speculate on what discoveries there may be around the corner.

We can, however, turn to the wider structures of civil society to record the growing ambition to develop and renew an approach to healing troubled minds that does not rely upon a chemical fix, but instead looks to work with personal relationships, human meaning, aspirations and values.

We have reviewed the early attempts to develop this new approach in the name of social psychiatry, and the ways that they gradually became dispersed – for good or ill – throughout society and social policy. We have explored two new frameworks – psychologically informed environments and enabling environments – that are now attempting to refresh our recognition of the importance of rebuilding the social fabric to address common mental health problems, with stress and trauma and psychiatric disorder now seen as part of a single continuum.

For a changing world, this book, as befits any writing in the early years of the 21st century, comes with a companion website, where the interested reader can now find further details, further examples, new research and policy digests and updates. This can be found at www.complextraumarecoveryenvironments.org.uk.

The future is, of course, uncertain. That is its strength. The future will not be determined by our genetic programming, but will be what we make it.

References

Ainsworth M, Blchar M, Waters E & Wall S (1978) *Patterns of Attachment: A psychological study of the strange situation.* Hillsdale, NJ: Erlbaum.

Alcoholics Anonymous (2007) How it works. In: *The Big Book Online* [online]. Alcoholics Anonymous World Services. Available at: www.alcoholics-anonymous.org.uk/bigbook/pdf/BigBook_chapt5.pdf (accessed January 2012).

Al-Khudhairy N (2000) The changing idea of community. In: S Tucker (ed) *A Therapeutic Community Approach to Care in the Community: Dialogue and dwelling.* London: Jessica Kingsley Publishers.

Alland A (1967) *Evolution and Human Behaviour.* London: Tavistock Publications.

Allen G & Smith I D (2010) The cross-party challenge: early intervention for children and families. *Journal of Children's Services* **5** (1) 4–8.

Ardrey R (1961) *African Genesis: A personal investigation into the animal nature and origins of Man.* New York: Atheneum.

Association of Directors of Adult Social Services (2008) *Mental Health into the Mainstream* [online]. London: ADASS. Available at www.adass.org.uk/index.php?option=com_content&view=article&id=287&Itemid=238 (accessed January 2012).

Ballat J & Campling P (2011) *Intelligent Kindness: Reforming the culture of healthcare.* London: Royal College of Psychiatrists.

Barrett J (2011) Sustainable organisation in health and social care: developing a 'team mind'. In: A Rubitel and D Reiss (Eds) *Containment in the Community: Supportive frameworks for thinking about antisocial behaviour and mental health.* London: Karnac.

Barton R (1976) *Institutional Neurosis* (3rd edition). Bristol: John Wright.

Baruch G & Treacher A (1978) *Psychiatry Observed.* London: Routledge and Kegan Paul.

Bateson P & Gluckman P (2011) *Plasticity, Robustness, Development and Evolution.* Cambridge: Cambridge University Press.

Batmanghelidjh C (2006) *Shattered Lives: Children who live with courage and dignity.* London: Jessica Kingsley Publishers.

BBC (2009) *Today* programme [online]. Available at: http://news.bbc.co.uk/today/hi/today/newsid_8235000/8235467.stm (accessed January 2012).

Becker S (1963) *Outsiders: Studies in the sociology of deviance.* New York: The Free Press.

Benjamin M, Savage S, Batmanghelidjh C (2009) *Developmental Traumatology: A review of the psychology, biology and neuroscience of childhood maltreatment.* London: Kids Company.

Bennett M & Hacker P (2003) *Philosophical Foundations of Neuroscience.* Oxford: Blackwell.

Berger P & Luckmann T (1966) *The Social Construction of Reality: A treatise on the sociology of knowledge.* New York: Anchor Books.

Bernal M, Haro J, Bernart S, Brugha T, de Graaf R, Bruffaerts R, Lepine J, de Giralomo G, Villagut G, Gasquet I, Torres J, Kovess V, Heider D, Neeleman J, Kessler R & Alonso J (2007) Risk factors for suicidality in Europe: results from the ESEMED study. *Journal of Affective Disorders* **101** (1–3) 27–34.

Berne E (1964) *Games People Play: The psychology of human relationships.* New York: Grove Press.

Berne E (1975) *What Do You Say After You Say Hello?* London: Corgi.

Better Regulation Executive (2009) *Striking the Right Balance* [online]. London: BRE. Available at: www.bis.gov.uk/assets/biscore/better-regulation/docs/10-578-striking-the-right-balance-bre-annual-review-2009.pdf (accessed January 2012).

Bion W (1961) *Experiences in Groups and Other Papers.* London: Brunner-Routledge.

Bonner A, Luscombe C, van den Bree M & Taylor P (2008) *The Seeds of Exclusion.* London: The Salvation Army.

Bowlby J (1973) *Attachment and Loss (Vol 2): Separation: Anxiety and anger.* London: Penguin.

Bowlby J (1980) *Attachment and Loss (Vol 3): Loss: Sadness and depression.* New York: Basic Books.

Bowlby J (1988) *A Secure Base: Clinical applications of attachment theory.* London: Routledge.

Box S (1971) *Deviance, Reality and Society.* London: Holt Rinehart and Winston.

Brown F (2003) *An Evaluation of the Concept of Play Value and its Application to Children's Fixed Equipment Playgrounds.* Unpublished PhD thesis: Leeds Metropolitan University.

Brown F & Webb S (2002) Playwork: An attempt at definition. In *Play Action* newsletter, Spring 2002 11–18.

Brown F & Webb S (2005) Children without play. *Journal of Education* **35** 139–158.

Bryce M (2007) Presentation at Integrated Living Network inaugural meeting. Wakefield: Northern Housing Consortium.

Buhrich N, Hodder T & Teesson M (2000) Lifetime prevalence of trauma among homeless people in Sydney. *Australian and New Zealand Journal of Psychiatry* **34** (6) 963–966.

Burkeman O Why everything you've been told about evolution is wrong *The Guardian*. **19 March**

Butler A & Hodos W (2005) *Comparative Vertebrate Neuroanatomy: Evolution and adaptation* (2nd edition). Hoboken, NJ: John Wiley & Sons.

Cabinet Office (2006) *Reaching Out: An action plan on social exclusion.* London: TSO. Available at: http://webarchive.nationalarchives.gov.uk/+/http://www.cabinetoffice.gov.uk/social_exclusion_task_force/publications/reaching_out.aspx (accessed January 2012).

Cahn E (2004) *No More Throw-Away People.* Washington, DC: Essential Books.

Capra F (1997) *The Web of Life: A new synthesis of mind and matter* (new edition). London: Flamingo.

Carey N (2011) *The Epigenetics Revolution: How modern biology is rewriting our understanding of genetics, disease and inheritance.* London: Icon Books.

Carroll R (2000) *An interview with Allan Schore* [online]. Available at: www.thinkbody.co.uk/papers/interview-with-allan-s.htm (accessed January 2012).

Centre for Mental Health (2011) *Briefing 43: A Place to Live: Securing stable accommodation for offenders with mental health problems.* London: Centre for Mental Health.

CHAIN (2009) *Profiling London's Rough Sleepers.* London: Broadway Homelessness and Support. Available at: www.broadwaylondon.org/CHAIN/CHAINResearch/ProfilingLondons RoughSleepers2009/main_content/ProfilingLondonsRoughSleepers SummaryReport.pdf (accessed January 2012).

Chaplin A (2011) Holistic Care Environmental Design: the future for dementia care. *Housing Care and Support* **14** (3) 91-97.

Charnwood Community Safety Partnership (2010) *Anti-Social Behaviour: The alternative incremental approach.* Charnwood: Charnwood Borough Council.

Choy A (1990) Winner's Triangle. *Transactional Analysis Journal* **20** (1) 40–46.

Christakis N & Fowler J (2009) *Connected: The surprising power of our social networks and how they shape our lives.* London: HarperCollins.

Clark D (1965) The Therapeutic Community: concept, practice and future. *British Journal of Psychiatry* **111** 947–954.

Clinard M & Meier R (2011) *Sociology of Deviant Behavior* (14th international edition). Florence, KY: Wadsworth.

Cockersell P (2010) Homelessness and Mental Health: adding clinical mental health interventions to existing social ones can greatly enhance positive outcomes. *Journal of Public Mental Health* **10** (2) 88–98.

Cockersell P (2011) More for Less? Using PIEs and recovery to improve efficiency in supported housing. *Housing Care and Support* **14** (2).

Cohen J & Stewart I (1994) *The Collapse of Chaos: Discovering simplicity in a complex world.* London: Penguin.

Connolly A, Cobb-Richardson P & Ball S (2008) Personality disorders in homeless drop-in center clients. *Journal of Personality Disorders* **22** (6).

Cooper Marcus C (2007) Healing gardens in hospitals. *Interdisciplinary Design and Research e-Journal, Design and Health* **1** (1).

Cozolino L (2002) *The Neuroscience of Psychotherapy: Building and rebuilding the human brain.* New York: Norton Professional.

Cozolino L (2006) The Neuroscience of Human Relationships: attachment and the developing social brain. *Psychotherapy in Australia* **12** (2).

Crawford M (2007) *Learning the lessons: A multi-method evaluation of dedicated community-based services for people with personality disorder.* London: Imperial College London/NCCSDO. Available at: www.sdo.nihr.ac.uk/files/project/83-final-report.pdf (accessed February 2012).

Crisis (2004) *Critical Condition: Homeless people's access to GPs: media brief.* London: Crisis. Available at: www.crisis.org.uk/downloads.php/102/GP_mediabrief.pdf (accessed January 2012).

Cromby J (2004) Between constructionism and neuroscience: the societal co-constitution of embodied subjectivity. *Theory and Psychology* **14** (6).

Cromby J (2005) Feelings and embodied subjectivity. In: V van-Deventer (Ed) *Proceedings of ISTP 2005.* Toronto: Captus Press.

Cullum S, O'Brien S, Burgess A, Booth J, Lant A & Catalan J (1995) Deliberate self-harm: The hidden population. *Health Trends* **27** (4) 130–132.

Daddow R & Broome S (2010) *Whole Person Recovery: A user-centred systems approach to problem drug use* [online]. London: Royal Society of Arts. Available at: www.thersa.org/projects/connected-communities/whole-person-recovery (accessed January 2012).

Damásio AR (1999) *The Feeling of What Happens: Body, emotion and the making of consciousness.* London: William Heinemann.

Damásio AR (2004) *Looking for Spinoza.* London: Vintage.

Damásio AR (2005) *Descartes' Error: Emotion, reason, and the human brain.* London: Penguin.

Daniels A (1970) The social construction of military psychiatric diagnoses. In: H Dreizel (Ed) *Recent Sociology 2.* London: MacMillan.

Dartington T (2010) *Managing Vulnerability: The Underlying Dynamics of Systems of Care.* London: Karnac.

Darton R, Bäumker T, Callaghan L & Netten A (2011) Improving housing with care choices for older people: The PSSRU evaluation of extra care housing. *Housing Care and Support* **14** (4).

De Bellis M (2005) The psychobiology of neglect. *Child Maltreatment* **10** (2) 150 –172.

De Board R (1978) *The Psychoanalysis of Organizations: A psychoanalytic approach to behaviour in groups and organizations.* London: Tavistock.

Dennett D (2003) *Freedom Evolves.* London: Alan Lane.

Department for Communities and Local Government (2006) *Places of Change: Tackling homelessness through the Hostels Capital Improvement Programme* [online]. London: CLG. Available: at www.communities.gov.uk/documents/housing/pdf/152564.pdf (accessed January 2012).

Department for Communities and Local Government (2009) *Guidance on Meaningful Interaction: How encouraging positive relationships between people can help build community cohesion.* London: CLG. Available at: www.communities.gov.uk/publications/communities/meaningfulinteraction (accessed January 2012).

Department for Communities and Local Government/National Mental Health Development Unit (2010) *Meeting the Psychological and Emotional Needs of People who are Homeless.* London: CLG/NMHDU. Available at www.nmhdu.org.uk/complextrauma (accessed January 2012).

Department of Health (2004) *The National Service Framework for Mental Health: Five years on* [online]. London: DoH. Available at: www.dh.gov.uk/en/Publicationsandstatistics/Publications/PublicationsPolicyAndGuidance/DH_4099120 (accessed January 2012)

Department of Health (2009a) *New Horizons: A shared vision for mental health.* London: DoH. Available at: www.dh.gov.uk/en/Publicationsandstatistics/Publications/PublicationsPolicyAndGuidance/DH_109705 (accessed January 2012).

Department of Health (2009b) *Recognising Complexity: Commissioning guidance for personality disorder services.* London: DoH. Available at: http://www.dh.gov.uk/prod_consum_dh/groups/dh_digitalassets/documents/digitalasset/dh_101789.pdf (accessed January 2012).

Department of Health (2010) *Healthy Lives, Healthy People: Our strategy for public health in England.* DoH: TSO. Available at: www.dh.gov.uk/en/Publichealth/Healthyliveshealthypeople/index.htm (accessed January 2012).

Department of Health (2011a) *Public Health Responsibility Deal.* London: DoH. Available at: www.dh.gov.uk/en/Publichealth/Publichealthresponsibilitydeal/index.htm (accessed January 2012).

Department of Health (2011b) *Response to the Offender Personality Disorder Consultation.* London: DoH. Available at: www.dh.gov.uk/prod_consum_dh/groups/dh_digitalassets/documents/digitalasset/dh_130701.pdf (accessed January 2012).

Department of Health/National Institute for Mental Health in England (2003a) *Personality Disorder: No longer a diagnosis of exclusion – policy implementation guidance for the development of services for people with personality disorder.* London: TSO.

Department of Health/National Institute for Mental Health in England (2003b) *Breaking the Cycle of Rejection: The personality disorder capabilities framework*. London: TSO.

Dictionary.com (2012) Trauma [online]. Available at: http://dictionary.reference/com/browse/trauma (accessed February 2012).

Dingwall R (1989) Some problems about predicting child abuse and neglect. In: O Stevenson (Ed) *Child Abuse: Pubic policy and professional practice*. Brighton: Wheatsheaf.

Dingwall R, Nerlich B & Hillyard S (2003) Biological determinism and symbolic interaction: hereditary streams and cultural roads. *Symbolic Interaction* **26** (4) 631–644.

DiPietro J, Kivlighan K, Costigan K, Rubin S, Shiffler D, Henderson J & Pillion J (2010) Prenatal antecedents of newborn neurological maturation. *Child Development* **81** 115–130.

Dockar-Drysdale B (1974) *Therapy in Child Care*. London: Longman.

Doidge N (2007) *The Brain that Changes Itself: Stories of personal triumph from the frontiers of brain science*. London: Penguin.

Dolan B & Coid J (1995) *Psychopathic and Antisocial Personality Disorders: Treatment and research issues*. London: Gaskell.

Edelmann G (1992) *Bright Air, Brilliant Fire: On the matter of the mind*. London: Penguin.

Elfer P, Goldschmied E & Selleck D (2003) *Key Persons in the Nursery: Building relationships for quality provision*. London: David Fulton.

Else P & Sturrock G (1998) The playground as therapeutic space: playwork as healing. In: A Skrupskelis (Ed) *Play in a Changing Society: Research, design, and application IPA / USA national conference*. Longmont, CO: Southern Early Childhood Association.

Fahmy E (2009) *Understanding the Risks of Social Exclusion Across the Life Course: Working age adults without dependent children*. Bristol: Social Exclusion Task Force/Cabinet Office. Available at: www.cabinetoffice.gov.uk/social_exclusion_task_force/life-course.aspx (accessed January 2012).

Fazel S, Khosla V, Doll H & Geddes J (2008) The prevalence of mental disorders among the homeless in Western countries: systematic review and meta-regression analysis. *PLoS Medicine* **5** (12).

Fisher K (2002) *It was magic!* Unpublished: Leeds Metropolitan University.

Fleck L (1979) *The Genesis and Development of a Scientific Fact*. Chicago: University of Chicago Press.

Folensbee R (2007) *The Neuroscience of Psychological Therapies*. Cambridge: Cambridge University Press.

Fonagy P (2004) Psychotherapy meets neuroscience: a more focused future for psychotherapy research. *Psychiatric Bulletin* **28** 357–359.

Foresight (2008) *Mental Capital and Well-being: Making the most of ourselves in the 21st century*. London: Foresight Mental Capital and Well-being Project.

Frey L, Beesley D & Newman J (2005) The relational health indices: Reanalysis of a measure of relational quality. *Measurement and Evaluation in Counseling and Development* **38** 153–163.

Fry S (2007) *The Ode Less Travelled: Unlocking the poet within*. London: Arrow Books.

Fulford K (2010) Presentation. Cambridge University Philosophy of Psychiatry Group.

Galderisi S & Mucci A (2000) Emotions, brain development, and psychopathology vulnerability. *CNS Spectrums* **5** (8) 44–48.

Gale J, Saftes E, Marrquez I & Espana B (2008) A psychological treatment programme for traumatised ex-military personnel in the UK. *Avances en psicología Latinoamericana* **26** (2) 119–234.

Gazzaniga M (2009) Edinburgh University Gifford Lecture series [online]. Available at: www.youtube.com/watch?v=dadT-14FkSY&list=PLEA9467E8E8D991AE&index=4&feature=plpp_video (accessed January 2012).

Gerhardt S (2004) *Why Love Matters.* London: Brunner-Routledge.

Gerhardt S (2010) *The Selfish Society.* London: Simon & Schuster.

Gladwell M (2005) *Blink: The power of thinking without thinking.* London: Penguin.

Glaser R & Kiecolt-Glaser J (1994) *Handbook of Human Stress and Immunity.* San Diego: Academic Press.

Goffman E (1959) *The Presentation of Self in Everyday Life.* London: Pelican.

Goffman E (1961) *Asylums: Essays on the social situation of mental patients and other inmates.* London: Pelican.

Goffman E (1971) *Relations in Public: Microstudies of the public order.* London: Penguin.

Goldacre B (2008) *Bad Science.* London: Fourth Estate.

Goleman D (1998) *Working with Emotional Intelligence.* London: Bloomsbury.

Greene Mintz T (2005) Relocation stress syndrome in older adults. *Social Work Today* **5** (6) 38. Available at: www.snapforseniors.com/portals/0/pdfs/relocationstress.pdf (accessed January 2012).

Greenfield S (2000) *The Private Life of the Brain.* London: Penguin.

Greig A & Taylor J (1999) *Doing Research with Children.* London: Sage.

Griffiths R (1988) *Community Care: Agenda for action.* London: DoH.

Griggs J, Whitworth A, Walker R, McLennan D & Noble M (2008) *Person or Place-Based Policies to Tackle Disadvantage? Not knowing what works.* York: Joseph Rowntree Foundation.

Groundswell (2010) *The Escape Plan* [online]. London: Groundswell. Available at: www.groundswell.org.uk/The_Escape_Plan_Report.pdf (accessed January 2012).

Gwadz M, Nish D, Leonard N & Strauss S (2007) Gender differences in traumatic events and rates of post-traumatic stress disorder among homeless youth. *Journal of Adolescence* **30** (1) 117–129.

Haigh R & Lees J (2008) Fusion TCs: divergent histories, converging challenges. *Therapeutic Communities* **29** (4).

Hansard (2011) *Parliamentary Debates,* House of Commons, February 28 2011, columns 53–54.

Harrison T (1999) A momentous experiment. In: P Campling P and R Haigh (Eds) *Therapeutic Communities: Past, present and future.* London: Jessica Kingsley Publishers.

Haw C, Hawton K & Casey D (2006) Deliberate selfharm patients of no fixed abode: a study of characteristics and subsequent deaths in patients presenting to general hospital. *Social Psychiatry and Psychiatric Epidemiology* **41** 918–925.

Hebb D (1949) *The Organization of Behaviour.* New York: John Wiley & Sons.

Henry J (1972) *Pathways to Madness.* London: Jonathan Cape.

Hill R & Brunsden V (2007) *Identifying the Needs of Relatives of Highlands and Islands Fire and Rescue Service Personnel.* Inverness: Highlands & Islands Fire & Rescue Service.

Hill R & Brunsden V (2009) Firefighters' experience of strike: an interpretative phenomenological analysis case study. *Irish Journal of Psychology* **30** (1) 97–113.

Hinshelwood R (1987) *What Happens in Groups.* London: Free Association.

Hinshelwood R & Manning N (Eds) (1979) *Therapeutic Communities: Reflections and progress.* London: Routledge and Kegan Paul.

Hinshelwood R & Skogstad W (Eds) (2000) *Observing Organisations: Anxiety, defence and culture in health care.* London: Brunner-Routledge.

Hirschhorn L (1997) *Reworking Authority: Leading and following in the post-modern organization.* Cambridge, MA: MIT Press.

HM Treasury (2010) *Total Place: A whole area approach to public services.* London: TSO. Available at: www.hm-treasury.gov.uk/psr_total_place.htm (accessed January 2012).

Hoggett P (2009) *Politics, Identity and Emotion.* London: Paradigm Publishers.

Homeless Link (2008, 2009, 2010, 2011, 2012) *Survey of Needs and Provision* (SNAP). London: Homeless Link. Available at www.homeless.org.uk/snap (accessed January 2012).

House of Commons (2010) *Government Response to the House of Commons Communities and Local Government Select Committee Report into the Supporting People Programme.* London: TSO. Available at www.communities.gov.uk/publications/housing/responsecommitteespprogramme?view=Standard (accessed January 2012).

Howarth I (2009) unpublished thesis (personal communication).

Huffington C & Armstrong D (Eds) (2004) *Working Below the Surface: The emotional life of contemporary organisations.* London: Karmac.

Hughes B (1996) *Play Environments: A question of quality.* London: PLAYLINK.

Illich I , Zola I, McKnight J, Caplan J & Shaiken H (1977) *Disabling Professions.* London: Marion Boyars.

Ingleby D (1981) *Critical Psychiatry: The politics of mental health.* London: Penguin.

Intelligent Space (2003) *The Impact of the Built Environment on Care Within A&E Departments* [online]. NHS Estates. Available at: www.intelligentspace.com/download/The%20Impact%20Of%20The%20Built%20Environment%20On%20Care%20Within%20A%20and%20E%20Departments.pdf (accessed January 2012).

Jacobs J, Horne-Moyer H & Jones R (2004) The effectiveness of critical incident stress debriefing with primary and secondary trauma victims. *International Journal of Emergency Mental Health* **6** (1) 5–14.

Jaques E (1953) On the dynamics of social structure. In: E Trist and H Murray (Eds) *The Social Engagement of Social Science, Vol 1: The socio-psychological perspective.* London: Free Association Books.

James O (2008) *The Selfish Capitalist: Origins of affluenza.* London: Vermilion.

James O (2009) Family under the microscope: how we react to stress is largely set in childhood – but it can be changed. *The Observer* **28 February**

James W (1902) *The Varieties of Religious Experience.* London & Bombay: Longmans, Green & Co.

Janssen E (Ed) (1980) *The Therapeutic Community: Outside the hospital.* London: Croom Helm for the Richmond Fellowship.

Johnsen S, Jones A & Rugg J (2008) T*he Experience of Homeless Ex-Service Personnel in London.* York: Centre for Housing Policy.

Johnson R (1981) *In search of the Enabling Environment* [online]. Planned Environment Therapy Trust. Available at: www.pettarchiv.org.uk/library/johnson1981.pdf (accessed January 2012).

Johnson R & Haigh R (2010) Social psychiatry and social policy for the 21st century: psychologically informed environments. *Mental Health and Social Inclusion* **14** (4) 30–35.

Johnson R & Haigh R (2011a) Social psychiatry and social policy for the 21st century: enabling environments. *Mental Health and Social Inclusion* **15** (1) 17–23.

Johnson R & Haigh R (2011b) Social psychiatry and social policy for the 21st century: new concepts for new needs: relational health. *Mental Health & Social Inclusion* **15** (2) 57–65.

Jones M (1968) *Beyond the Therapeutic Community: Social learning and social psychiatry.* New York: Yale University Press.

Jordan J (2001) A relational-cultural model: healing through mutual empathy. *Bulletin of the Menninger Clinic* **65** (1) 92–103.

Kahnemann D (2011) *Thinking, Fast and Slow.* London: Allen Lane.

Kandel E (1998) A new intellectual framework for psychiatry. *American Journal of Psychiatry* **155** (4) 457–69.

Karpman S (1968) Fairy tales and script drama analysis. *Transactional Analysis* **7** 26.

Keats H, Cockersell P, Haigh R, Johnson R & Maguire N (2012) *Psychologically informed services for homeless people*. In development.

King's Fund (2011) Childhood maltreatment & depression [online]. London: King's College London. Available at: www.kcl.ac.uk/newsevents/news/newsrecords/2011/08August/Childhood-maltreatment-long-term-depression-risk-poor-response-treatment.aspx.

Kytle B & Ruggie, JG (2005) *Corporate Social Responsibility as Risk Management: A model for multinationals.* Cambridge MA: John F Kennedy School of Government, Harvard University. Available at www.hks.harvard.edu/m-rcbg/CSRI/publications/workingpaper_10_kytle_ruggie.pdf (accessed January 2012).

Laing RD (1966) *The Divided Self.* London: Pelican.

Laing RD (1967) *The Politics of Experience and the Bird of Paradise.* London: Penguin.

Laing RD & Esterson A (1964) *Sanity, Madness and the Family.* London: Pelican.

Lansley A (2009) *Working with Business to Improve Public Health: Conclusions of the responsibility deal working group.* London: Public Health Commission.

Lawlor D & Webb L (2009) An interview with Isabel Menzies Lyth with a conceptual commentary. *Organisational and Social Dynamics* **9** (1).

Lawrence L & Barber G (2004) Debriefing in the fire service. *Counselling at Work* **winter 2004** 11–13.

LeDoux J (1998) *The Emotional Brain: The mysterious underpinnings of emotional life.* London: Weidenfeld & Nicholson.

LeDoux J (2002) *Synaptic Self: How our brains become who we are.* New York: Viking.

Lees J (2004) *A Culture of Enquiry: Research evidence and the therapeutic community.* London: Jessica Kingsley Publishers.

Lemert E (1951) *Social Pathology: A systematic approach to the theory of sociopathic behavior.* New York: McGraw-Hill.

Levitin D (2007) *This is Your Brain on Music.* London: Atlantic.

Lewin K (1948) *Resolving Social Conflicts.* New York: Harper and Row.

Liebling A & Arnold H (2004) *Prisons and their Moral Performance: A study of values, quality, and prison life.* Oxford: Oxford University Press.

Liotti G (2007) 'Disorganised attachment and therapeutic relationships with people in shattered states'. Conference presentation, John Bowlby Memorial Conference, London.

Lyons M (2006) *National Prosperity, Local Choice and Civic Engagement: A new partnership between central and local government for the 21st century* [online]. London: Lyons Inquiry. Available at: www.lyonsinquiry.org.uk/ (accessed January 2012).

MacIntyre A (1985) *After Virtue* (2nd edition). London, Duckworth.

Maguire N, Johnson R, Vostanis P, Keats H & Remington R (2010) *Homelessness and Complex Trauma: A review of the literature* [online]. University of Southampton. Available at: www.personal.soton.ac.uk/nm10/Complex_Trauma.doc (accessed January 2012).

Main T (1946) The hospital as a therapeutic institution. *Bulletin of the Meninger Clinic* **10** 66–70.

Malenbaum S, Keefe F, Williams A, Ulrich R & Somers T (2009) Pain in its Environmental Context: Implications for designing environments to enhance pain control. *Pain* **134** (3) 241–244.

Manning N (2001) Psychiatric diagnosis under conditions of uncertainty: personality disorder, science, and professional legitimacy. In: J Busfield (Ed) *Rethinking the Sociology of Mental Health* (pp76–94). Oxford: Blackwell Publishing.

Marcus G (2008) *Kluge: The haphazard construction of the human mind.* London: Faber and Faber.

Marmot M (2009) *Strategic Review of Health Inequalities in England post 2010.* Available at: www.marmotreview.org (accessed January 2012).

Marmot M & Wilkinson R (2003) *Social Determinants of Health: The solid facts (second edition).* Denmark: World Health Organization. Available at: www.euro.who.int/__data/assets/pdf_file/0005/98438/e81384.pdf (accessed January 2012).

Martin E (Ed) (2010) *Concise Medical Dictionary* (8th Edition). Market House Books.

Maslow A (1971) *The Farther Reaches of Human Nature.* New York: Viking Press.

Matza D (1964) *Delinquency and Drift.* New York: John Wiley and Sons.

Matza D (1969) *Becoming Deviant.* New Jersey: Prentice-Hall.

Mead G (1934) *Mind, Self and Society: From the standpoint of a social behaviourist.* Chicago: University of Chicago Press.

Menzies I (1990) Social systems as a defence against anxiety: an empirical study of the nursing service of a general hospital. In: E Trist and H Murray (Eds) *The Social Engagement of Social Science, Vol 1: The socio-psychological perspective.* London: Free Association Books.

Middleton R (2008) *Brokering Reality: A review of service provision in Leeds for homeless people with personality disorder / complex needs.* Leeds: Leeds Partnerships/NHS Foundation Trust.

Milliband E (2011) 'The Big Society: A cloak for the small state *Independent on Sunday* **13 February**.

Milton A (2010) speech at King's Fund seminar, July 2010 [online]. Podcast available at: www.kingsfund.org.uk/events/past_events_catch_up/public_health_a_new.html (accessed January 2012).

Moncrieff J (2007) *The Myth of the Chemical Cure*. Basingstoke: Palgrave Macmillan.

Morris D (1966) *Men and Apes*. London: Hutchinson.

Murphy T, Burley A & Worthington H (2002) *Homelessness and Personality Disorder*. Edinburgh: Lothian Primary Care NHS Trust.

Nanni V, Uher D & Danese A (2011) Childhood maltreatment predicts unfavorable course of illness and treatment outcome in depression: a meta-analysis. *American Journal of Psychiatry* doi: 10.1176/appi.ajp.2011.11020335

National Social Inclusion Programme (2009) *Vision and Progress*. London: NSIP.

Nature (2010) *The Psychopathic Brain* [online]. NeuroPod podcasts available at: www.nature.com/neurosci/neuropod/index-2010-03-29.html (accessed January 2012).

NICE (2009a) *Antisocial Personality Disorder (CG77)*. London: NICE. Available at: http://guidance.nice.org.uk/CG77.

NICE (2009b) *Borderline Personality Disorder (BPD) (CG78)*. London: NICE. Available at: www.nice.org.uk/CG78 (accessed February 2012).

Norman J (2010) *The Big Society*. Buckingham: UBP.

Northern Housing Consortium (2009) *Enabling Environments: Feedback on the draft standards* [online]. Sunderland: NHC. Available at: www.northern-consortium.org.uk/assets/policy/09%2005%20enabling%20environments%20-%20nhc%20response.pdf (accessed January 2012).

Obholzer A and Zagier Roberts C (Eds) (1994) *The Unconscious at Work: Individual and organizational stress in the human services*. London: Routledge.

Oliver M (1990a) *The Politics of Disablement*. Basingstoke: MacMillan.

Oliver M (1990b) *The Individual and Social Models of Disability: People with established locomotor disabilities in hospitals*. Leeds: Leeds University. Available at www.leeds.ac.uk/disability-studies/archiveuk/Oliver/in%20soc%20dis.pdf (accessed January 2012).

O'Shea M (2005) *The Brain: A very short introduction*. Oxford: Oxford University Press.

Panksepp J (1998) *Affective Neuroscience*. Oxford: Oxford University Press.

Patton P (2008) One world, many minds: intelligence in the animal kingdom. *Scientific American Mind* **December 2008/January 2009**.

Pearce B (2004) *Using CMM: The co-ordinated management of meaning*. Woodside, CA: Pearce Associates.

Perry B (2005) *Maltreatment and the Developing Child: How early childhood experience shapes child and culture*. In: A Cunningham (Ed) The Margaret McCain Lecture Series. Canada: The Centre for Children & Families in the Justice System.

Perry B, Pollard R, Blakley T, Baker W & Vigilante D (1995) Childhood trauma, the neurobiology of adaptation, and 'use-dependent' development of the brain: how states become traits. *Infant Mental Health Journal* **16** 271–291.

Pert C (1998) *Molecules of Emotion*. New York: Simon and Shuster.

Pinker S (1997) *How the Mind Works*. London: Penguin.

Prior L (1993) *The Social Organization of Mental Illness*. London: Sage.

Public Health Agency of Canada (2006) *The Human Face of Mental Health and Mental Illness in Canada*. Ottowa: Minister of Public Works and Government Services Canada. Available at: www.cpa.ca/cpasite/userfiles/Documents/Practice_Page/Human_Face_2006_EN.pdf (accessed January 2012).

Putnam R (2000) *Bowling Alone: The collapse and revival of American community.* New York: Simon & Schuster.

Rappoport R (1960) *Community as Doctor.* London: Tavistock.

Rees S (2009) *Mental Health in the Adult Single Homeless Population: A review of the literature.* London: Public Health Resource Unit/Crisis. Available at: www.crisis.org.uk/data/files/publications/Mental%20health%20literature%20review.pdf (accessed January 2012).

Regier D, Farmer M & Rae D (1990) Comorbidity of mental disorders with alcohol and other drug abuse. *Journal of the American Medical Association* **264** (25).

Ridley M (2003) *Nature via Nurture: Genes experience and what makes us human.* London: Fourth Estate.

Rose S (2005) *Lifelines: Life beyond the gene* (revised edition). London: Vintage.

Rose S (2006) *The 21st Century Brain.* London: Vintage.

Rose S, Bisson J, Churchill R & Wessely S (2002) *Psychological Debriefing for Preventing Post Traumatic Stress Disorder* (Cochrane Review). Cochrane Database of Systematic Reviews 2002, Issue 2, Article Number: CD000560. DOI: 10.1002/14651858.CD000560

Roth A & Fonagy P (2004) *What Works for Whom? A critical review of psychotherapy research* (2nd edition). New York: Guilford Press.

Royal College of Psychiatrists (2010) *No Health Without Public Mental Health: The case for action.* London: RCPsych. Available at: www.rcpsych.ac.uk/policy/policyandparliamentary / parliamentandpublicaffairs/neilspages/publicmentalhealth.aspx (accessed January 2012).

Ryan R & Deci E (2000) Self-determination theory and the facilitation of intrinsic motivation, social development and well-being. *American Psychologist* **55** (1) 68–78.

Sanderson L & Brunsden V (2011) *Help Seeking in the Military.* Nottingham: Nottingham Trent University.

Sapolsky R (1998) *Why Zebras Don't Get Ulcers: A guide to stress, stress-related disease, and coping* (2nd edition). New York: W H Freeman.

Sayce L (2000) *From Psychiatric Patient to Citizen: Overcoming discrimination and social exclusion.* Basingstoke: Palgrave.

Scanlon C & Adlam J (2006) Housing 'unhoused minds': inter-personality disorder in the organisation? *Housing, Care and Support* **9** (3) 9–14.

Scheff T (1999) *Being Mentally Ill: A sociological theory* (3rd edition). New York: Aldine de Gruyter.

Schore A (1994) *Affect Regulation and the Origin of the Self: The neurobiology of emotional development.* New Jersey: Lawrence Erlbaum Associates.

Shur E (1971) *Labelling Deviant Behaviour: Its sociological implications.* New York: Harper & Row.

Searle J (2007) *Freedom and Neurobiology: Reflections on free will, language, and political power.* New York: Columbia University Press.

Seivewright N & Daly C (1997) Personality disorder and drug use: a review. *Drug and Alcohol Review* **16** 235–250.

Selye (1975) Confusion and controversy in the stress field. *Journal of Human Stress* **1** (2) 37–44.

Sempik J, Hine R & Wilcox D (Eds) (2010) *Green Care: A conceptual framework: A report of the working group on the health benefits of green care, COPST Action 866, Green Care in Agriculture.* Loughborough: Centre for Child and Family Research, Loughborough University.

Shapiro E & Carr A (1991) *Lost in Familiar Places: Creating new connections between the individual and society.* New Haven: Yale University Press.

Shepherd G, Boardman J & Slade M (2008) *Making Recovery a Reality.* London: Centre for Mental Health.

Shotter J (1993) *Cultural Politics of Everyday Life.* Buckingham: Open University Press.

Siegel D (2011) *The Mindful Therapist.* New York: W W Norton & Co.

Singleton N, Meltzer H & Gatward R (1998) *Psychiatric Morbidity among Prisoners in England and Wales.* London: Office for National Statistics.

Slater L (2004) Monkey love. *The Boston Globe* **21 March**. Available at: www.boston.com/news/science/articles/2004/03/21/monkey_love/?page=full (accessed January 2012).

Social Care Institute for Excellence (2011) *Short-Notice Care Home Closures: A guide for local authority commissioners* [online]. London: SCIE. Available at: http://www.scie.org.uk/publications/homeclosures/ (accessed January 2012).

Social Exclusion Unit (2002) *Reducing Re-Offending by Ex-Prisoners.* London: SEU. Available at: http://webarchive.nationalarchives.gov.uk/+/http://www.cabinetoffice.gov.uk/media/cabinetoffice/social_exclusion_task_force/assets/publications_1997_to_2006/reducing_summary.pdf (accessed January 2012).

Social Exclusion Unit (2004) *Mental health and Social Exclusion.* London: Office of the Deputy Prime Minister. Available at: www.socialinclusion.org.uk/publications/SEU.pdf (accessed January 2012).

Solomon M & Siegel D (2003) *Healing Trauma.* New York: W W Norton & Co

Stanton A & Schwartz M (1954) *The Mental Hospital: A study of institutional participation in psychiatric illness and treatment.* New York: Basic Books.

Stewart A, Steiman M, Cauce A, Cochran B, Whitbeck L & Hoyt D (2004) Victimization and post traumatic stress disorder among homeless adolescents. *Journal of the American Academy of Child and Adolescent Psychiatry* **43** (3) 325–331.

Stewart K (1992) *The York Retreat in the Light of the Quaker Way.* York: Erbor Press.

St Mungo's (2010) *Client Needs Survey*. London: St Mungo's.

St Mungo's (2011) *Lifeworks: How an innovative psychotherapy project is helping homeless people in their recovery*. London: St Mungo's. Available at: www.mungos.org/homelessness/publications/latest_publications_and_research (accessed January 2012).

Sudnow D (1967) *Passing On: The social organization of dying.* New Jersey: Prentice Hall.

Suomi S & Harlow H (1971) Monkeys without Play. In: J Bruner, A Jolly and K Sylva (Eds) (1976) *Play: Its role in development and evolution.* New York: Basic Books.

Sutton-Smith B (1997) *The Ambiguity of Play.* Cambridge, MA: Harvard University Press.

Taylor K & Sharpe L (2008) Trauma and post-traumatic stress disorder among homeless adults in Sydney. *Australian and New Zealand Journal of Psychiatry* **42** (3) 206–213.

Teicher M, Andersen S, Polcari A, Anderson C, Navalta C & Kim D (2003) The neurobiological consequences of early stress and childhood maltreatment. *Neuroscience and Biobehavioral Reviews* **27** (1–2) 33–44.

Timms P & Fry A (1989) Homelessness and mental health. *Health Trends* **21** 70–71.

Tooby J & Cosmides L (1992) The psychological foundations of culture. In: J Barkow, L Cosmides and J Tooby (Eds) *The Adapted Mind: Evolutionary psychology and the generation of culture.* New York: Oxford University Press.

Torgerson S, Kringlen E & Cramer V (2001) The prevalence of personality disorders in a community sample. *Archives of General Psychiatry* **58** (6) 590–596. Available at: http://archpsyc.ama-assn.org/cgi/content/abstract/58/6/590 (accessed February 2012).

Trew B (2011) The boy who refused to riot. *Evening standard* **5 September.**

Trist E & Murray H (Eds) (1990) *The Social Engagement of Social Science Vol 1: The social-psychological perspective.* London: Free Association Books.

Tyrer P (2008) Personality disorder and public mental health. *Clinical Medicine* **8** (4) 1–5.

Tyrer P & Kramo K (2007) Nidotherapy in practice. *Journal of Mental Health* **16** (1) 117–129.

Vaglum P, Friis S, Jorstad J, Karterud S & Lorentzen S (1982) From a panacea to a special treatment method. *International Journal of Therapeutic Communities* **3** (1).

van der Kolk B, Pynoos R, Cicchetti D, Cloitre M, D' Andrea W, Ford J, Lieberman A, Putnam F, Saxe G, Spinazzola J, Stolbach B, Teicher M (2009) Proposal to Include a Developmental Trauma Disorder Dignosis for Children and Adolescents in DSM-V [online]. Available at: www.cismai.org/ScaricaFile.aspx?ID=65&T=1 (accessed February 2012).

Verheul R (2001) Co-morbidity of personality disorders in individuals with substance use disorders. *European Psychiatry* **16** 274–282.

Webb S & Brown F (2003) Playwork in adversity: working with abandoned children. In: F Brown (Ed) *Playwork: Theory and practice.* Buckingham: Open University Press.

Welch S (2002) *Personality Disorders and Substance Misuse* [online]. Available at: www.csip.org.uk/silo/files/pd-and-ddpdf.pdf (accessed January 2012).

Whittington D (2011) Wrenching open the doors of perception. *Attachment: New directions in psychotherapy and relational psychoanalysis* **5** 15–38.

Widdershoven G, McMillan J, Hope T & Van der Scheer L (Eds) (2008) *Empirical Ethics in Psychiatry.* Oxford: Oxford University Press.

Wilkinson R (2006) *The Impact of Inequality: How to make sick societies healthier.* London: Routledge.

Wilkinson R & Pickett K (2009) *The Spirit Level: Why more equal societies almost always do better.* London: Allen Lane.

Williamson P & Allman J (2011) *The Human Illnesses: Neuropsychiatric disorders and the nature of the human brain.* Oxford: Oxford University Press.

Wilson E (1975) *Sociobiology: The new synthesis.* Cambridge, MA: Harvard University Press.

Winnicott D (1965) *The Maturational Processes and the Facilitating Environment.* London: Karnac Books.

Woodhouse D & Pengelly P (1991) *Anxiety and the Dynamics of Collaboration.* Aberdeen: Aberdeen University Press.

World Health Organization (1953) *Expert Committee on Mental Health: 3rd report.* Geneva: WHO. Available at: http://whqlibdoc.who.int/trs/WHO_TRS_363.pdf (accessed January 2012).

Young Foundations (2009) *Sinking and Swimming: Understanding Britain's unmet needs.* London: Young Foundations.

Zeanah C & Shah P (2005) *Attachment and its impact on child development: Comments on van IJzendoorn, Grossmann and Grossmann, and Hennighausen and Lyons-Ruth* [online]. Centre of Excellence for Early Childhood Development. Available at: www.child-encyclopedia.com/documents/Zeanah-ShahANGxp.pdf (accessed January 2012).

Futher reading

For the website that expands and discusses many of the subjects in this book, see www.complextraumarecoveryenvironments.org.uk